The Economics of Health

The Economics of Health

Donald J. Meyer

2016

W.E. Upjohn Institute for Employment Research
Kalamazoo, Michigan

Library of Congress Cataloging-in-Publication Data

Names: Meyer, Donald J., editor.
Title: The economics of health / [edited by] Donald Meyer.
Description: Kalamazoo, Michigan : W.E. Upjohn Institute for Employment Research, 2016. | Includes index.
Identifiers: LCCN 2016005812| ISBN 9780880994620 (pbk. : alk. paper) | ISBN 0880994622 (pbk. : alk. paper) | ISBN 9780880994637 (hardcover : alk. paper) | ISBN 0880994630 (hardcover : alk. paper)
Subjects: LCSH: Medical economics.
Classification: LCC RA410 .E2873 2016 | DDC 338.4/73621—dc23
LC record available at http://lccn.loc.gov/2016005812

W.E. Upjohn Institute for Employment Research
300 S. Westnedge Avenue
Kalamazoo, Michigan 49007-4686

Cover design by Alcorn Publication Design.
Index prepared by Diane Worden.
Printed in the United States of America.
Printed on recycled paper.

Contents

Acknowledgments vii

1 **Introduction** 1
Donald J. Meyer

2 **We Have Met Our Enemies and They Are Us** 7
Charles E. Phelps

3 **Do Medical Care and Self-Care Compete or Complement in Health Production?** 35
Donald J. Meyer

4 **Payment Reform and "Bending the Curve"** 51
John H. Goddeeris

5 **The Potential Effects of the Affordable Care Act on Disability Insurance and Workers' Compensation** 81
Marcus Dillender

6 **The Economic Challenges of the Community Living Assistance Services and Supports Act** 103
Edward C. Norton

7 **The Role of Private Health Insurance in the Medicare Program** 117
M. Kate Bundorf

Authors 143

Index 145

About the Institute 155

Acknowledgments

The chapters in this book are based on presentations made at the forty-eighth annual Werner Sichel Economics Lecture Series, hosted by the Department of Economics during the 2012–2013 academic year on the campus of Western Michigan University. The series is made possible through financial support of the W.E. Upjohn Institute for Employment Research and Western Michigan University (WMU). It is named for Dr. Werner Sichel, who retired in 2005 following 45 years of teaching at WMU.

1 Introduction

Donald J. Meyer
Western Michigan University

Securing good health is vitally important for each of us individually, as well as for our society as a whole. In fact, maintaining an acceptable level of health is necessary to adequately function in our daily lives. Health brings us happiness with the ability to feel good, to be pain-free, and to enjoy life. We yearn to have a rich, fulfilling life, and good health is the vehicle for being able to do so; it allows us to function productively in our jobs and reduces our number of sick days, which results in additional income and a higher standard of living.

The importance of good health extends to our overall economy as well. Health care makes up about 17 percent of our national economy and thus greatly affects our macroeconomy. Rising health care costs have presented challenges for the national budget, and incentive issues due to health uncertainty and asymmetric information have important market implications for our health economy. Furthermore, the obesity epidemic in our country is an alarming situation, contributing to deteriorating health, premature death, and escalating health care costs.

The passage and recent implementation of the Patient Protection and Affordable Care Act (ACA) has been extremely controversial. Important components of this historic act include the contentious personal mandate, the newly established state exchanges, and Medicaid expansion. Although the purpose of this book is not to critique the ACA, several chapters in this volume do evaluate how specific aspects of the ACA affect our economy.

When addressing or modeling health, economists typically posit a utility function $U(C,H)$, where consumers derive utility from consuming various goods and services (C), as well as from the level of health (H) they possess. Health can be thought of as an economic good that consumers work to acquire, similar to a stock or consumer durable, such as an automobile or a refrigerator. We need to model utility over time and consider investments made to our health stock over our lifetimes. Utility maximization requires a trade-off between investing our scarce time and money into the acquisition of health or the consumption of other goods and services.

A significant aspect of the market for health is that the health level to be consumed *must* be produced by the same individual—that is, none of the health we wish to consume can be purchased as such in the marketplace. This is a very atypical situation in our economy; generally, consumers do not produce the good, they purchase it in the marketplace. It is similar to a family farmer who can eat only the vegetables that he grows himself. This leads to less specialization in production and more generalization.

Thus it becomes important to consider how one best produces an acceptable level of health for present and future consumption. Two significant inputs into the production of health are medical care and lifestyle choice or self-care. Doctor visits, medical procedures, and pharmaceuticals help improve our health; many of us receive these services through health insurance coverage that we purchase or obtain through our employers. Personal choices, such as the amount of physical exercise we get, our alcohol consumption, and calorie intake also influence our health. Other inputs that affect our health include education level, random health shocks, and the environment in which we live.

Uncertainty pervades over health determination, as our health status even one or two years into the future is highly unknown or uncertain. Our attitude toward the risk is very important in determining how we manage it. Buying insurance is one response to facing a random loss due to illness or disease. Health insurance is central to one's insurance portfolio, but other types of insurance can help in the events of becoming disabled, getting hurt on the job, or requiring assisted living. One can also invest in self-protection or self-insurance through a healthier lifestyle, including eating better food, exercising, and limiting alcohol and tobacco consumption.

Health markets are also heavily subject to situations of asymmetric information—when one party knows more information than another party about some health aspect. Adverse selection, nonrepresentative risk pools, and death spirals can result when individuals know more about their health risks than the insurance companies. Moral hazard, or a change in behavior upon having insurance, can cause people to take on more health risks or overpurchase health insurance. The agency problem involves the challenge of hiring doctors or other health professionals to investigate our health issues and make decisions that are in our best interests.

This book contains six chapters that address various aspects of health. Charles E. Phelps begins the volume with "We Have Met Our Enemies and They Are Us." This provocative title refers to the fact that many of us in the United States do not make good lifestyle choices. Phelps cites a study that shows that poor choices regarding tobacco usage, eating, activity, and alcohol consumption make up the leading causes of death in the United States. He suggests working to improve the educational system, as education rates are generally positively correlated with making healthier lifestyle choices.

Phelps finds a direct relationship between medical spending and both income and life expectancy, but an inverse relation between medical spending and infant mortality. The extent to which the United States is a major outlier is surprising; we spend far more on medicine than any other country and have health results that are far from what our health expenditures would predict.

Chapter 3, "Do Medical Care and Self-Care Compete or Complement in Health Production?," by Donald J. Meyer, focuses on two of the primary input categories in one's health production function, medical care and self-care. He asks whether these two input types function more closely as substitutes or complements. Loosely speaking, are medical care and self-care more often used in combination with each other, or do individuals more likely choose one over the other? Meyer reviews arguments for each of these ideas, the complementarity relations that competing risk models indicate and the basic substitution effect based on relative prices and productivities.

Meyer first notes the two basic definitions in neoclassical production of two inputs having a complement or substitute relation. He then argues that this issue is more appropriately viewed in the context of significant uncertainty, a primary characteristic of the health setting. A common response to decision making under uncertainty is the attainment of market insurance and/or the practice of undertaking self-insurance or self-protection, two categories of self-care. Meyer reviews much of the literature in which researchers have debated whether these uncertainty responses are used more in a complementarity or substitution manner.

He recognizes and discusses the close link that exists between medical care and health insurance, thus enabling a more enriched definition of complements and substitutes between medical care and self-care in the health context. He then reviews three articles that have examined whether medical care and self-care are better described as complements or substitutes, and he offers his own opinions as well.

The next three chapters deal with some aspect of the Patient Protection and Affordable Care Act (ACA). John H. Goddeeris's chapter is entitled "Payment Reform and 'Bending the Curve.'" The "bending the curve" phrase has been attributed to President Barack Obama, who in 2009 said, "It is important for us to bend the cost curve . . . because the system we have right now is unsustainable . . ." This refers to the challenge of keeping health care costs under control and limiting the rate of annual increase of the costs. Goddeeris considers one such possible curve—health care costs as a percentage of gross domestic product—which has been growing consistently over the last 50 years and has reached a level of about 17 percent.

Goddeeris then addresses ways in which health care providers are paid, which he argues is a critical component of bending the curve. He examines aspects of paying for output rather than inputs, managed competition, and bundling by episode. Goddeeris argues for a more global payment method regarding some specific defined population versus a traditional fee-for-service plan. He discusses in detail the idea of an Accountable Care Organization and how this might better function in terms of incentives for receiving care and controlling costs.

Marcus Dillender's chapter is entitled "The Potential Effects of the Affordable Care Act on Disability Insurance and Workers' Compensation." Disability insurance covers people who are unable to work for over a year due to health concerns, and workers' compensation insurance pays medical costs for people who get injured while working on the job. These two types of insurance that relate to how the risk of health deterioration affects one's earning or income potential are sometimes overlooked by individuals who are concerned about addressing health risks in general.

The two main sections of the chapter examine basic program information for disability insurance and workers' compensation and how the ACA affects the likelihood of filing a claim for these types of insurance. Dillender also considers how the ACA may affect our health system more generally, which can then indirectly spill over to the two types of insurance.

Edward C. Norton considers the issue of long-term care in his chapter, "The Economic Challenges of the The Community Living Assistance Services and Supports Act." The CLASS Act was a major component of the original ACA, but it ultimately was not supported and was struck from the act that passed in 2010. It would have created a market for long-term care with a number of interesting features. He reviews the expenditure needs of the typical elderly individual and notes that long-term care offers the greatest variance in out-of-pocket expense and thus is the riskiest issue facing the elderly.

Norton discusses why the CLASS Act was dropped from the ACA legislation, and he suggests that the proposed act faced many significant economic challenges. One challenge was adverse selection and moral hazard, present in all insurance markets but even more pronounced in the elderly long-term care market. Another challenge was inflation risk—claims made for long-term care insurance are often made decades into the future, when the purchasing power of your benefit amount is subject to years of inflationary erosion. Norton also suggests that the long-run viability of the program was in question due to the financial instability of funding the program long term.

Chapter 7, by M. Kate Bundorf, is entitled "The Role of Private Health Insurance in the Medicare Program." Bundorf introduces her topic by laying out the basic Medicare system in the United States. Parts A and B make up traditional Medicare originating in 1965 and cover hospital, physician, outpatient, and other standard forms of health care services. Part D was added under the Medicare Modernization Act of 2003 and adds outpatient prescription drug benefits.

Bundorf then focuses on two forms of private insurance that interact with the Medicare system. The first is Medicare Part C, or Medicare Advantage, which allows beneficiaries to enroll in a private plan that replaces traditional Medicare (parts A and B). The second is Medigap, a private policy that supplements existing Medicare. Medigap policies reduce deductibles and cover copays, reducing personal cost liability. This tends to accentuate moral hazard, as Bundorf notes. She evaluates the two different programs and how they have both increased Medicare spending over the years and then discusses how future Medicare reform may be differentially affected by the two plans.

Good health is a characteristic that is crucial to all of us individually and collectively as a country. The United States is challenged in its world ranking in health statistics, which is likely to become an even larger challenge as its population ages over the next few decades (Phelps discusses this in Chapter 2). Education in general appears to be an ally for good health and for becoming better informed about our health system, and it helps reduce uncertainty and aids in better decision making for all of us. The chapters in this volume contribute to this end and are indicative of the type of health research work that is needed.

2
We Have Met Our Enemies and They Are Us

Charles E. Phelps
University of Rochester

HEALTH CARE SPENDING AND OUTCOMES—AN INTERNATIONAL PERSPECTIVE

Many critics (and even some proponents) of the U.S. health care system note two things: 1) we spend a lot of money on health care, far more than any other country in the world; and 2) we don't get the best health outcomes in return.

Let's first look at health care spending. Figure 2.1 shows U.S. spending per capita against per capita gross domestic product (GDP), with other countries' incomes and spending standardized to U.S. dollars using appropriate exchange rates. These data (from the Organisation for Economic Co-operation and Development [OECD]) show a remarkable pattern—as per capita GDP rises, medical spending rises at a very predictable rate (at about 1.5 × the rate of per capita GDP).[1] One remarkable feature is how close to the best-fit line we can find countries with incredibly different health care systems, including Great Britain (with a socialized health care system), Canada (with a socialized health *insurance* system but private production of health care itself), Germany and Japan (with private production but mixed insurance systems), Sweden (with county-level government health plans), and Australia (with a system not much different from that in the United States). All of these nations, despite the differing roles of government in their health care structure, have essentially the same spending on health care once taking into account the predictable differences due to per-capita GDP differences.

Figure 2.1 Income and Medical Spending in OECD Countries

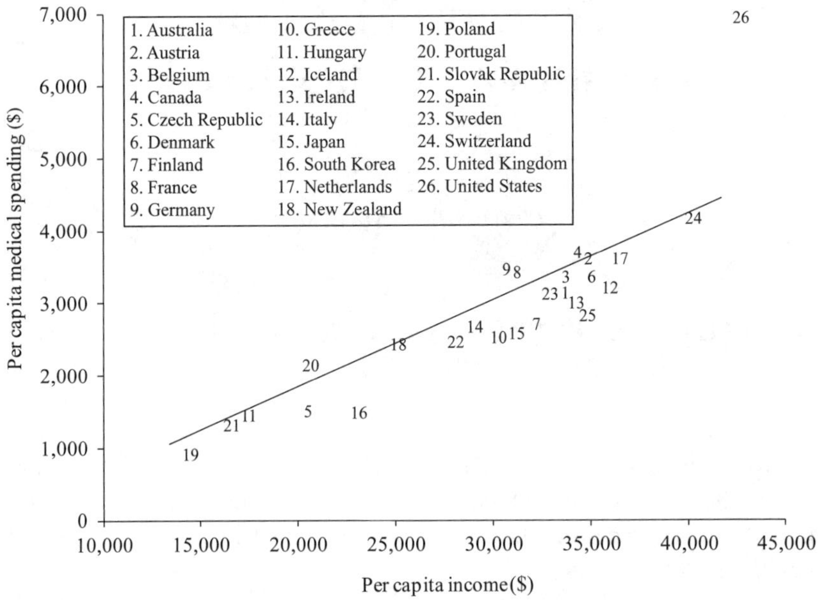

SOURCE: Author's calculations using OECD data.

The United States looms as an outlier on the regression line fitted from other nations' data points. We are wealthier than other countries, but our medical spending far outstrips the level predicted from the best-fit regression line. We have demonstrably profligate spending habits for health care.

When looking at our health outcomes, a gloomier picture emerges. The United States again sits as an outlier but clearly in the wrong direction. Figure 2.2 shows how life expectancy at birth and per capita medical spending correlate. The pattern is not nearly as tight as that between medical spending and per capita GDP, but a recognizable (albeit fuzzy) link exists between medical spending and health outcomes. In general, countries that spend more have better longevity. Japan looms large as a happy outlier—it has the highest life expectancy in the world, despite relatively middle-of-the-road medical spending. Genetics likely plays a role, but dietary choices have a large effect. When first-generation Japanese move to Hawaii, they maintain their Japanese longevity if they

Figure 2.2 Life Expectancy and Medical Spending for OECD Countries

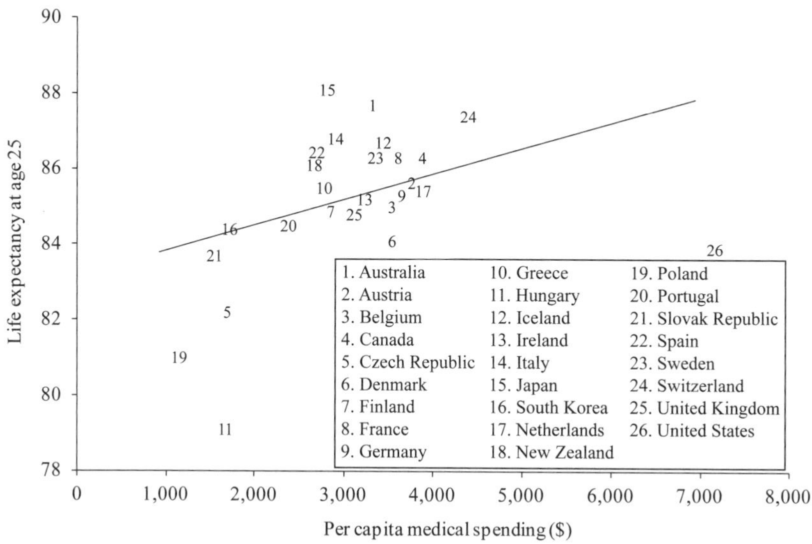

SOURCE: Author's calculations using OECD data.

retain traditional Japanese dietary patterns, but if they acquire American dining habits, they also acquire American mortality rates (Kolonel, Hinds, and Hankin 1980; Tanabe, n.d.).

A clearer picture emerges when looking at infant mortality rates, as shown in Figure 2.3. Here the pattern is crisper than with life expectancy at birth, but once again we can see that more medical spending generally reduces perinatal mortality; the United States has far-worse outcomes than the best-fit line would predict. We in fact have perinatal mortality rates normally associated with countries with about one-third of our medical care spending rate, including Portugal and the former Warsaw Pact state of the Slovak Republic. The United States has about triple the infant mortality rate that the best-fit regression line would predict.

This gloomy portrait of our health care system has many root causes, some of which I explore later in this chapter. Before moving to that, however, we need a quick peek into the future. Here's a hint: Things will get worse, not better.

Figure 2.3 Infant Mortality vs. Medical Spending in OECD Countries

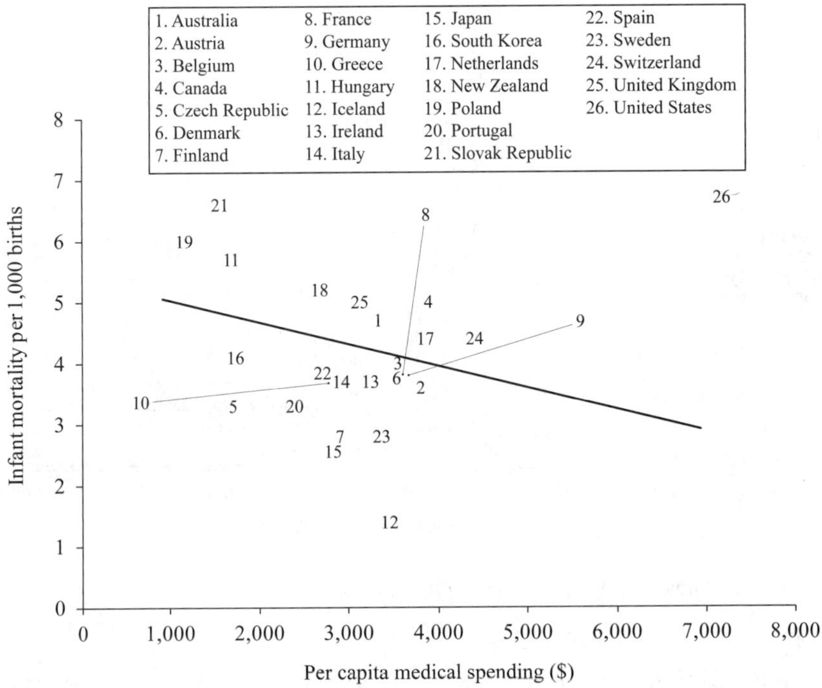

SOURCE: Author's calculations using OECD data.

THE LIGHT AT THE END OF THE TUNNEL IS A TRAIN COMING AT US

Demographers show the age mix of a country's population using what they used to call "population pyramids." The horizontal bars in these graphs represent age groups, older as one moves up the pyramid. The left side shows males, the other shows females. They are called pyramids because they are wide at the base (youngest age groups) and narrower at the top (older age groups), reflecting increased mortality as we get older.

Over time, however, these pyramids can change shape, and in very predictable ways, depending on how long people live and the birth rate that brings new entrants into the population (babies). Figures 2.4A, 2.4B, and 2.4C show current projections from the U.S. Census Bureau for the population that embeds predictions about future age-specific mortality rates and also birth rates. The 1950 chart shows a typical pyramid, pinched in at the bottom, however, both for losses to military deaths and lower fertility rates during World War II. It also shows the baby boom at the end of the war (the wide band for 0–4-year-olds) that has important consequences for later years' forecasts. Now, skip ahead to the 2000 pyramid. These data are also known with certainty. The baby boom of the 1945–1950 era (and nearby cohorts) has now moved into middle age, and the pyramid shows a hefty "middle-aged spread," not unlike that of a lot of the actual baby boomers. Note also the lop-sided and enlarged age mix at the top. The pyramid no longer comes to a point, and it is very decidedly female. Women outlive men in the United States by about five years, mostly owing to the effects of earlier cigarette smoking. Very large fractions of our nursing home populations are women who were widowed many years earlier in their lives.

Skipping ahead to 2025 and 2050 involves making projections about the future, which demographers do using models to forecast age-specific mortality rates and also to forecast birth rates. The 2025 forecasts show an increasingly top-heavy age distribution, and by 2050, the pyramid turns into a shape like a graduation cap—it has far more people in the 80+ age group than any other five-year interval, and the ratio of working age to retired has become very unfavorable. Some pundits now call this the "Silver Tsunami."

Health care spending rises rapidly with the number of chronic conditions (see Figure 2.5), which are closely linked to age as our bodies wear out faster and faster. It does not take a complex computer program to tell us that the combination of an aging population and the increased rate of medical spending with age and its associated increase in chronic conditions will inevitably lead to increasingly higher health care spending. Unless something dramatically changes, U.S. spending could easily exceed one-fourth—perhaps even one-third—of GDP on health care by 2050. Spending rates will inevitably rise over time. Our only meaningful goal is to somehow cut down the rate of growth. Health care pundits call this "bending the curve." Subsequent sections in this chapter discuss ways to do this that lie outside the realm of health care reform.

Figure 2.4 Age Profiles for U.S. Population, 1950–2050

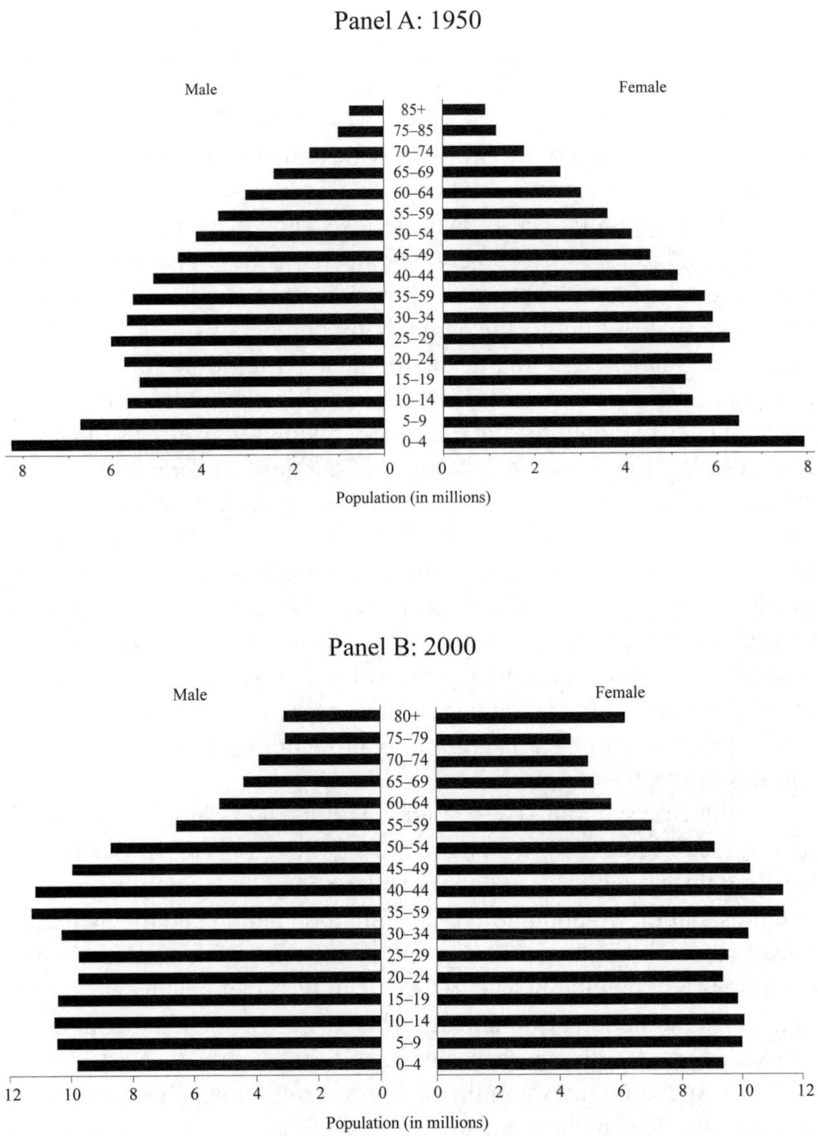

Figure 2.4 (continued)

Panel C: 2025

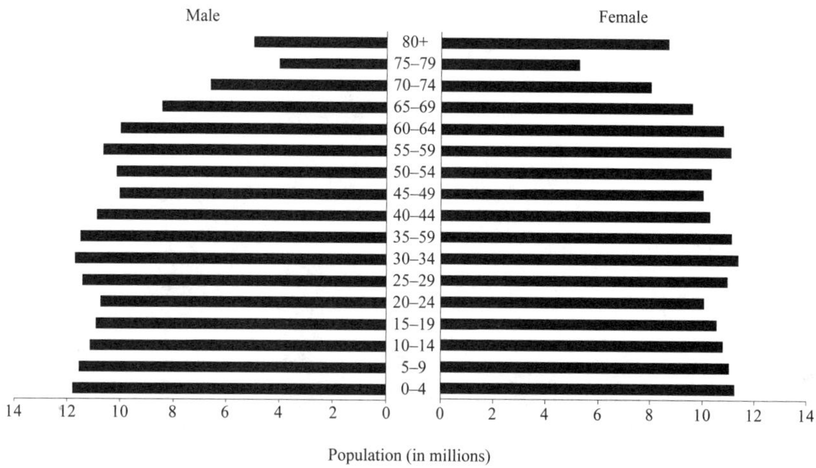

Panel D: 2050

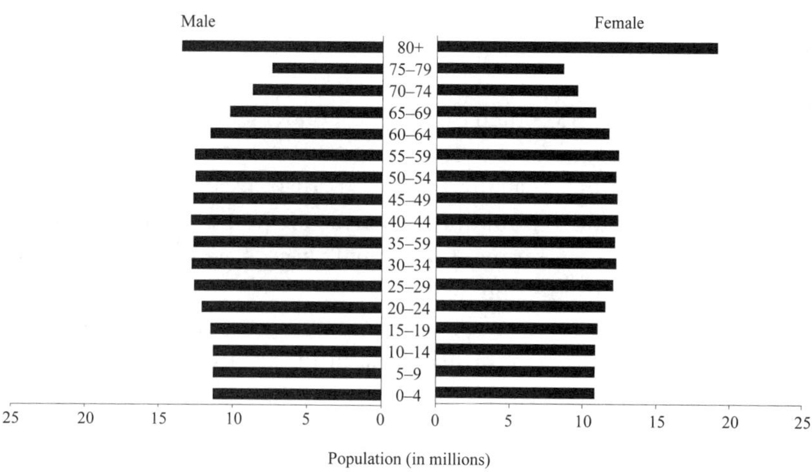

SOURCE: U.S. Census Bureau.

Figure 2.5 Average Health Care Spending per Capita, by Number of Chronic Conditions, 2010

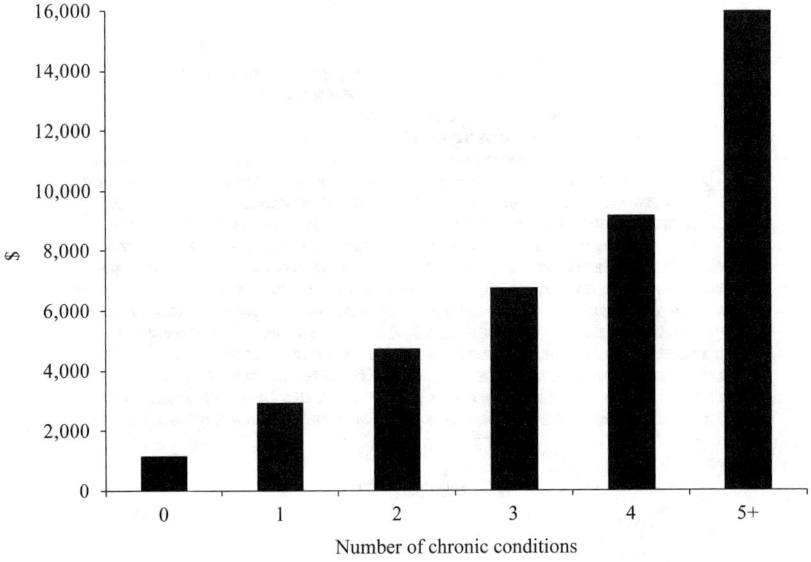

SOURCE: 2010 Medical Expenditure Panel Survey.

We Are Our Own Worst Enemy

Most people in the United States don't understand the true causes of death and the large medical costs that arise as we try to stave it off. We read about and witness deaths from heart disease, cancer, and stroke, but these are just the natural consequences of the true causes of death. The brutal truth is that, for many, personal choices are often the primary true causes of our illness and death.

In a powerful study combining epidemiologic studies and mortality data, McGinnis and Foege (1993) look at the excess mortality arising from various lifestyle choices and combine that with death certificate data to come to an astonishing conclusion: the leading cause of death in the United States is our own behavior. To see how this works, suppose that last year 1,000 people died of Disease X—the death certificate would show that disease is the cause. Now, suppose that of those 1,000 people, 750 were tobacco users. Since only about 25 percent of the U.S. population smokes, tobacco users are overrepresented among those who died of Disease X by a factor of three. If the disease were unrelated to tobacco use, we would expect to find only 250 tobacco users among the 1,000 who died of Disease X, but we actually saw 750. So, we attribute 500 excess deaths from Disease X to tobacco.

Now, do the same thing for other diseases, such as lung cancer, many other types of cancer, chronic obstructive pulmonary disease, heart attack, heart failure, and stroke, and then add up the excess deaths attributed to tobacco. When you finish that list, tobacco, it turns out, is the leading cause of death in the United States. Mokdad et al. (2004) redid the original study 10 years later using data from 2000. The results, shown in Figure 2.6, are quite stunning. These nine causes of death account for about half of all deaths, and most of these—surely we would include tobacco, diet/inactivity, alcohol, motor vehicle accident, firearms, sexual behavior, and illicit drug use—are wholly matters of human behavior and choice. One could easily include toxic agents in the list as well (primarily consequences of air and water pollution), but that may be more of a societal issue rather than an individual choice. Let's look at the most important of these in more detail.

Figure 2.6 Actual Causes of Death in the United States, 2000

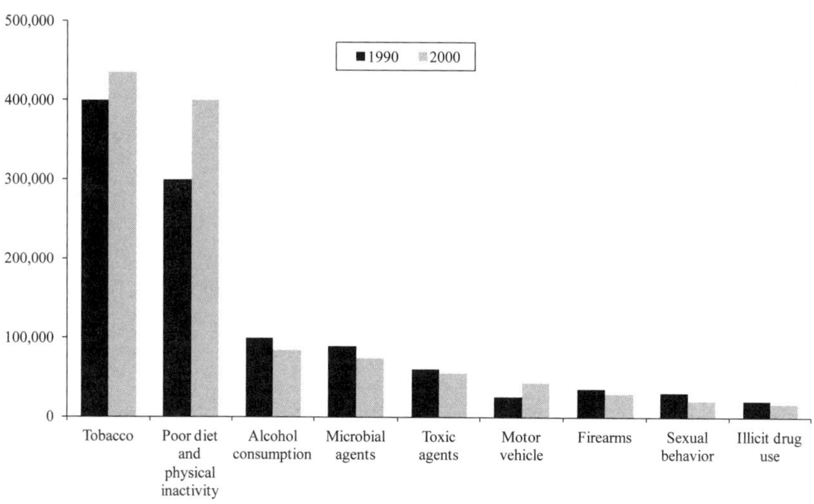

SOURCE: Data from Mokdad et al. (2004).

Tobacco

Despite the enormous mortality burden from tobacco, the problem is actually lessening. Some of the decline comes from improved cancer treatment (arising in part from NIH research), but much of it is attributed to reduced smoking rates. Americans now smoke at about half the rate they did in 1965. Figure 2.7 shows per-adult cigarette consumption patterns from 1900 to 2010.

Many things converged to cause this sea change. Most importantly, a 1964 report from the U.S. surgeon general greatly shifted patterns of tobacco use over time and spurred many cultural and legal changes (U.S. Department of Health, Education, and Welfare 1964).[2]

Warning labels appeared on cigarette packages. Television ads for tobacco were banned, and antismoking ads were aired instead. Local and state governments banned smoking in restaurants. Smoking was no longer permitted on airplanes and in most airports. Cigarette taxes

Figure 2.7 Cigarettes Smoked per Year in the United States

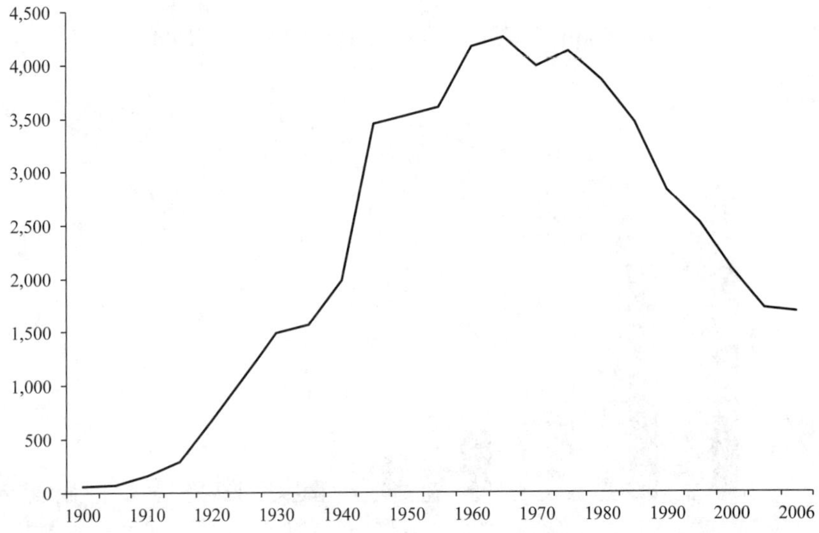

SOURCE: Warner (1989) and author's calculations using data from the U.S. Centers for Disease Control and Prevention.

increased dramatically. The smoking culture changed. Before the surgeon general's report, cigarette smoking was a standard Hollywood sign of sophistication. Ayn Rand praised smoking extensively in *The Fountainhead* (1943). People smoked in restaurants, in homes, in the park, on trains, in hotel rooms—everywhere, both public and private. Now the public perception of smoking is quite different: it is widely considered a sign of ignorance and/or irrational behavior.

Over time, many antismoking laws have been passed, and many jurisdictions (both in the United States and worldwide) have made smoking illegal not only in most indoor public settings but in many outdoor places as well. And it is certainly considered ill-mannered for people to light up in any private home without permission. All of these cultural and legal changes came from one source—a government report. Now, instead of nearly half of the population smoking cigarettes, fewer than 20 percent do so. By convening the committee to write this report, Dr. Luther Terry, the then surgeon general, may have saved more lives than any other physician in history.

Eschewing the Fat?

The next causes of death I address here are poor diet and lack of exercise. It is perhaps politically incorrect to say this, but the evidence seems clear: fat kills. Being overly skinny is also unhealthy, but that's generally not the weight problem that affects most people.

To understand the definition of overweight, we need to define the body mass index (BMI), which is widely used to measure obesity, defined (in metric measurements) as weight (in kilograms) divided by height (in meters) squared.[3]

Standard ranges for adults are as follows: normal, 22–24; overweight, 25–29; obese, 30–35; and morbidly obese, over 35. An increasing proportion of the U.S. population falls into the obese and morbidly obese categories. There is a national epidemic of obesity, yet it draws far less attention than do many far less dangerous epidemics of various "bugs."

First, let's look at the data on the growth in obesity. Figure 2.8 shows data from regular surveys of the U.S. population beginning in 1960. The percent of adults classified as "overweight" (BMI between 25 and 30) stays essentially flat at about a third of the population throughout this

Figure 2.8 Obesity Trends in the United States

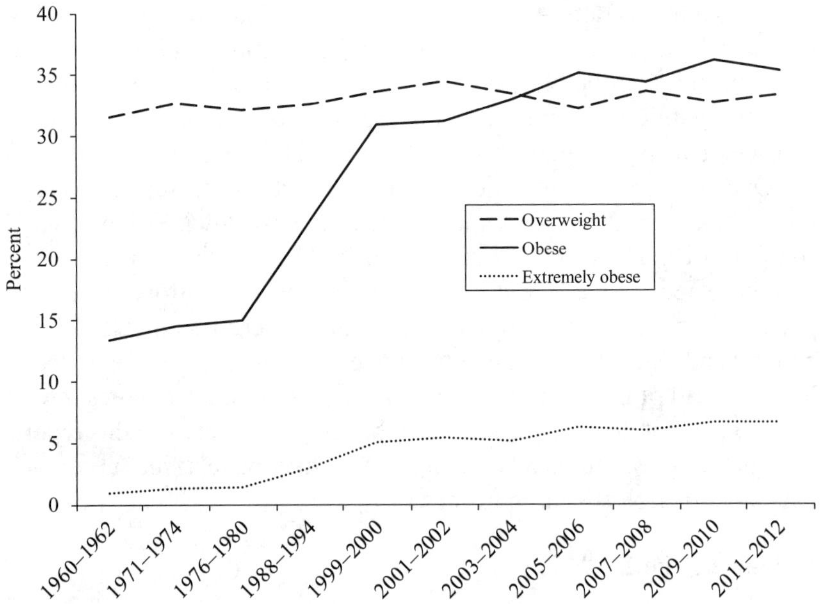

SOURCE: U.S. Department of Health and Human Services.

half century, but those who are obese (BMI between 30 and 40) begins to climb rapidly after about 1980. The combined group of "obese" and "extremely obese" grew from under 15 percent in 1960 to 42 percent in the most recent years—a tripling of the rate of obesity and now almost half of the adult population. Similar data (not shown) reveal a similar pattern for adolescents and children.

Now let's look at the effects of obesity on health and consider the ultimate indicator of health: survival rates. Figure 2.9 shows the relative risk of death (in any single year) by BMI category, separately for men and women, using the lowest-risk group as 1. Thus, a relative risk of 1.5 means a person has a 50 percent greater chance of dying than a person in the best BMI group.[4]

The width of the bars shows the statistical imprecision (which gets worse as the number of people in each group shrinks), but the midpoint of each bar shows the average relative risk.

Figure 2.9 Body Mass Index (BMI) and All-Cause Mortality

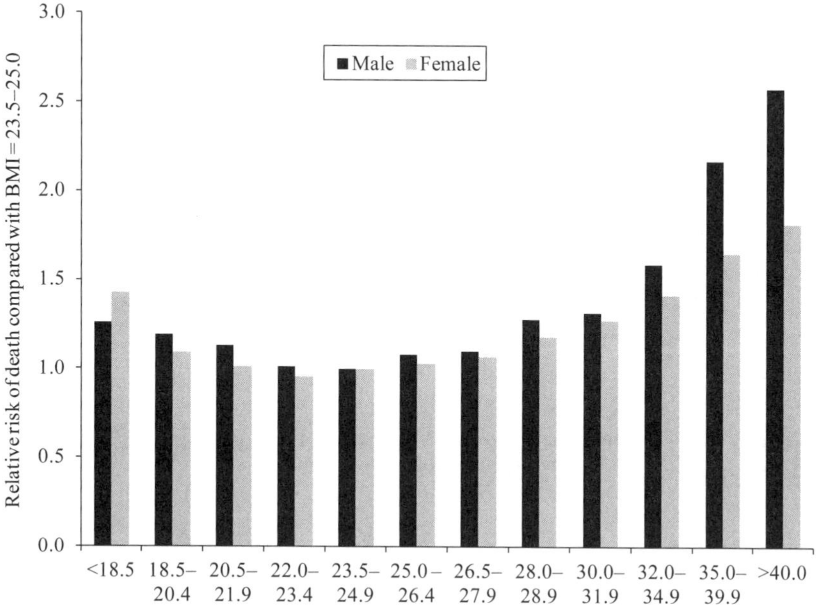

SOURCE: Calle et al. (1999).

For both men and women, the best survival rates appear in the groups with a BMI of 23.5–24.9. The relative risk climbs both for people with lower and higher weight than this "most-protective" BMI. But, as the data in Figure 2.8 show, our problem in the United States is not an epidemic of underweight, but rather the opposite—obesity.

Obesity causes many disorders that degrade the quality of life, and its associated diseases reduce people's ability to do many enjoyable things in life. It increases the risk of hypertension (half of all hypertension comes from obesity), heart disease, numerous cancers, sleep apnea, abdominal hernias, gout, and varicose veins. For people who are obese, the risk of diabetes triples, and with diabetes comes other ailments such as vision problems, skin breakdown, and further risk of heart disease. Bringing body weight into normal ranges (BMI of about 23–25) can eliminate about 40 percent of all heart disease.

Stewart, Cutler, and Rosen (2009) calculate the average quality of life people report in different age groups by BMI category and smoking status, because of all the chronic conditions brought about by smoking and obesity, both have systematic effects on the quality of life people report (see Figure 2.10). Where 100 is perfect health, quality scores fall as BMI rises, and they also are worse for smokers than for nonsmokers. At almost every age, an obese smoker reports about 80 percent of the quality of life as the normal-weight nonsmoker.

Obesity costs a lot of money. The Centers for Disease Control pegged the costs of obesity-related diseases at nearly $150 billion per year in 2008 (Finkelstein et al. 2009). The average obese person uses about $1,500 more—approximately 40 percent—per year in medical services than a person of normal weight. This affects tax dollars through the funding of Medicare and Medicaid, and the costs of our private insurance go up in the same way because obese people pay the same premium as nonobese people.

Alcohol

To understand the health effects of alcohol, we need to bring two concepts into the picture. First, the real health problems come with heavy drinking and binge drinking.[5] Heavy drinking is known to increase the risk of various cancers, liver disease (particularly cirrhosis), and heart disease. However, almost ironically, regular moderate alcohol use seems to have a series of health-protective aspects, especially with regard to heart disease, more so when the alcohol of choice is wine, and especially so for some red wines with high levels of particularly beneficial complex chemicals.[6] A large study of Danish adults (Grønbaek et al. 2000) finds that heavy drinkers of distilled spirits had about double the cancer risk of nondrinkers, but those who drank wine moderately (not heavy or binge) had a 20 percent lower all-cause mortality rate and almost cut the risk of heart disease in half (compared with nondrinkers).

We Are Fighting the Wrong Drug War

The official war on drugs focuses on substances such as marijuana, cocaine, and heroin, but those drugs account for less than 1 percent of

Figure 2.10 Quality of Life by Smoking and BMI Status

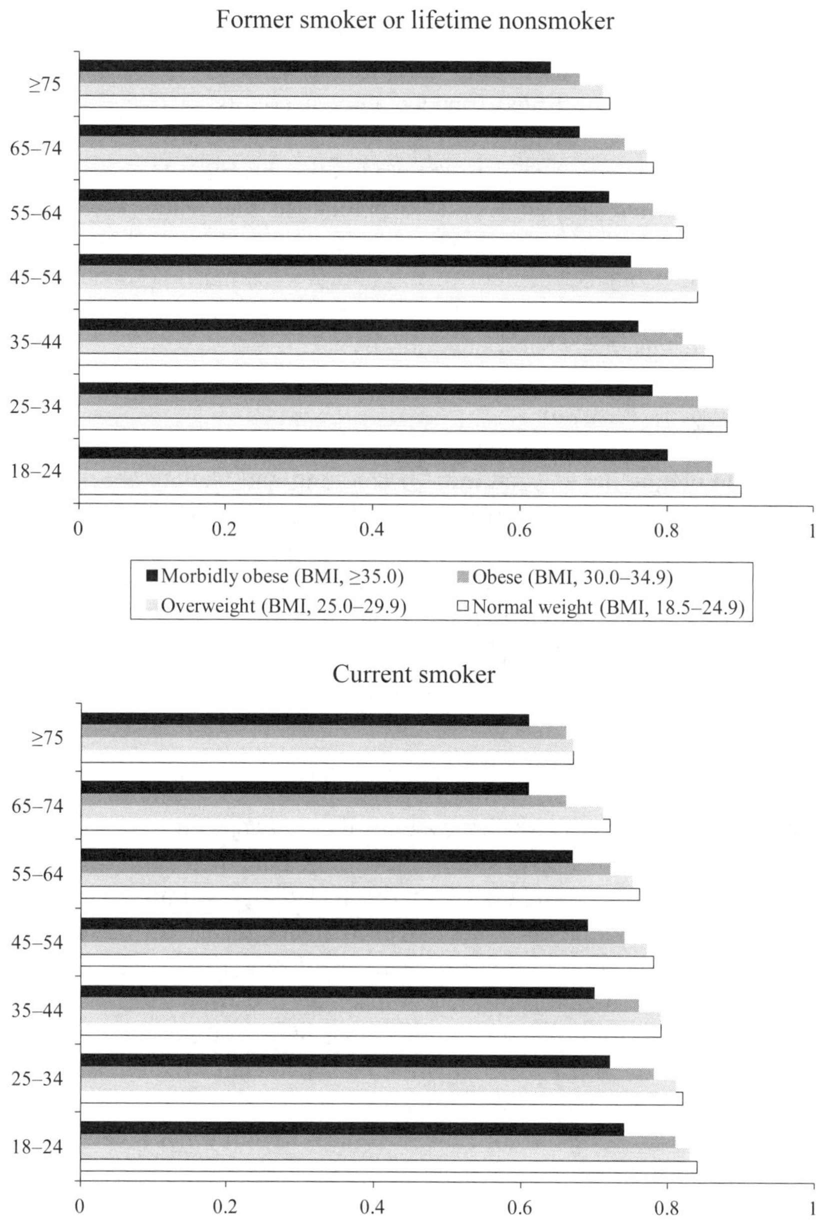

SOURCE: Stewart, Cutler, and Rosen (2009).

all deaths in the United States. Tobacco, on the other hand, causes 18 percent of the deaths in our country every year. Alcohol adds another 3.5 percent, for a total of 21.5 percent for these two legal drugs. This means that tobacco and alcohol account for 30 times as many deaths each year as do illicit drugs. Tobacco alone accounts for over 25 times the number of deaths as illicit drugs.

If we were to count obesity as an addictive problem (as some people do), we could add another 16.6 percent to the deaths associated with addictive behavior—tobacco, calories, alcohol, and illicit drugs. Together they total 39 percent of the nation's deaths. The conclusion seems obvious: we are fighting the wrong drug war. The big health issue isn't illicit drugs, it's tobacco and obesity.

The European Paradox

Some people have asked me, "If smoking and obesity are the real issues, why don't the Europeans (or the Japanese) have health costs higher than ours, since they smoke at much higher rates than we do?" It is an excellent question for which I do not have a conclusive answer; I have only a few ideas to help think about the issue.

First, if people in Europe or Japan smoked less, the smoking/risk data almost guarantee that their health costs would fall. Second, we are just beginning to reap the benefits of the gradual decline in smoking rates in the United States.

Further, the Europeans mostly have implicit or explicit rationing mechanisms in their health care systems that put caps on costs in a way that selectively saves costs due to smoking. Part of this comes from the observation that smokers die early in their lives, thus precluding their incurring some other potentially expensive diseases (Manning et al. 1989). But in most European societies, deaths that would involve expensive hospitalization in the United States, cancer treatment, and intensive care do not get treated the same way. For example, half of all deaths in the United States involve intensive care, whereas in Great Britain, only 1 in 10 does (Wunsch et al. 2009).

Intensive care unit use for cancers is three to four times higher in the United States than in Britain and eight times higher for strokes, two of the main "death certificate" causes of death of smokers.

Finally, many Europeans regularly follow what is now known as the “Mediterranean” diet, which emphasizes plant-based foods, such as fruits and vegetables, whole grains, legumes, and nuts. In a large-scale randomized trial in which people were assigned to follow either the Mediterranean diet or a low-fat diet, two important things emerged (Estruch et al. 2013). First, the Mediterranean diet improved health and longevity (versus the low-fat diet). Second, because our bodies seem to be “wired” otherwise, people didn’t adhere to the low-fat diet, so the study became a comparison of the Mediterranean diet versus a standard diet. The study had such large differences in the primary outcomes of cardiac- or stroke-related death that the research was stopped early because it became unethical to continue to forbid the low-fat group from switching to the Mediterranean diet.

THE LONG-RUN “FIX”

Complicated problems seldom have simple solutions. The burdens that our lifestyle choices place on our lives and our health care costs cannot be solved with a magic bullet. However, there are some practical ways to help fix these problems.

Focus on the Underlying Health Risks

To address the problem, we almost surely need a massive investment in public and private resources to find biologically based measures to help people alter their behaviors, most notably tobacco use and poor food choices. Urging people to change their ways will not suffice. We have had modest success in reducing smoking through public awareness, restricting smoking in public, higher taxes on cigarettes, and more readily available smoking cessation products.

We have had far less success in reducing obesity. The epidemic proportions of increasing obesity attest to this problem. So also do the countless ads for weight-loss programs, some based on caloric control, planned menus, diets low (or high) in carbohydrates, low-fat diets, balanced diets, and group support. Some products hint at effective weight loss from various natural substances, usually with a warning such as "results not typical" next to the before and after photos of someone who appears to have lost a lot of weight. Very few FDA-approved medications are available for weight loss. This highlights the problem: in order to claim that a drug helps people lose weight, the FDA requires scientifically valid proof. Most weight-loss programs can't sustain the losses people achieve initially. Herbal and natural remedies are not subject to FDA approval; thus, claims made about these diet aids are not as controlled as are those for prescription drugs. The FDA has approved several weight-loss drugs, one of which (by prescription) affects the brain's hunger signals. The first over-the-counter weight-loss drug was approved in 2007 and works by blocking the body's ability to absorb fat. Therein lies the rub: what goes in must get burned or come out. Those who take this drug and eat fatty foods often get a very sudden reminder that they have recently consumed fat.[7]

For the dangerously obese (defined as having a BMI > 40), a relatively new approach called bariatric surgery shrinks or bypasses the stomach so that the person feels full after eating less.[8] This works well for some people, but it has potential side effects such as acid reflux (with overeating), nausea, and vomiting.

There is an old joke among economists: two economists are walking down the street, and one sees a $100 bill lying in the gutter. As he leans over to pick it up, the other economist admonishes him, "If it were a real $100 bill, somebody would have picked it up already." Diet aids are like that—if there were one that really worked and kept weight off forever, it would dominate the market. Instead, we see herbs and spices, various nonprescription drugs, acupressure and acupuncture, group therapy, individual counseling, exercise programs, meditation, prayer groups, and surgical interventions. Americans annually spend $33 billion on weight-loss products, about $150 per adult per year, yet we still gain weight (collectively) at an astonishing rate. The lack of success provided by existing weight-control methods tells us that we need something new.

Radically Restructure NIH Research Priorities

Managing the adverse health consequences (death, illness, injury, pain, work loss, productivity loss) and associated medical costs of poor lifestyle choices will require a massive investment in basic research to better understand the causes, treatments, and prevention of these key addictive and behavioral choices—primarily tobacco and obesity, but alcohol abuse as well. In 1965, President Lyndon Johnson declared war on heart disease, cancer, and stroke, securing massive increases in funding through the various National Institutes of Health (NIH) to study the causes and cures of these diseases. That effort has paid great dividends in reductions of death and morbidity from these diseases. The funding priorities of the NIH today show just how far behind we are on the issues of tobacco and obesity. The NIH budget provides $30 billion total for all NIH endeavors. Of this, $5 billion goes to the National Cancer Institute (NCI), $3 billion to the National Heart, Lung and Blood Institute (NHLBI), and $1.6 billion for the National Institute of Neurological Disorders and Stroke (NINDS), adding up to almost a third of the NIH budget.

By contrast, NIH funding for the National Institute on Alcohol Abuse and Alcoholism rests at $400 million. The National Institute on Drug Abuse received $1 billion in funding in 2009. We have no national institute to deal with tobacco addiction or obesity. Although some of the NCI, NHLBI, and NINDS funds go toward prevention research, these agencies' research agendas are dominated with "cure" approaches.

I suggest that one of the best ways to reduce federal and private health care spending over the next 50 years would be a massive investment in federal research to find effective ways to eliminate tobacco use and excessive caloric intake (obesity). This cannot succeed if done half-heartedly. In 2003 the NIH formed an obesity task force that has published and regularly updated a strategic plan to deal with obesity. It discusses cross-cutting research and emphasizes the need to deal with behavioral modification, pharmacologic approaches, and surgical approaches. Astonishingly, these reports have no mention of budgets. Not a single word appears to suggest allocation of funds toward reducing obesity. Nobody is in charge. An old dictum (in a particularly inept choice of metaphors in this case) says, "If you assign two people to feed a dog, it will starve to death." That is where the NIH is with obesity.

In 2000, one study looked at every grant issued by the NIH (across all institutes) to estimate the research funding directly focused on tobacco and nicotine use (Hughes and Liguori 2000). The 1995 total (their most recent year of data) showed $92 million in dedicated research on this issue, less than one-half of 1 percent of the NIH extramural budget.

Therein sits the stark contrast: we spend about a third of the NIH budget on curing heart disease, cancer, and stroke, and we spend less than half of 1 percent on prevention associated with tobacco use. Exactly how much the NIH is currently devoting to obesity research remains unknown, but the fact that its strategic plan for dealing with the problem utters not a single word about budgetary commitment speaks volumes.

Improve K–12 Education

We have another important tool at our disposal—education. I don't mean provision of specific information about healthy lifestyles, but rather general K–12 education and postsecondary education. According to the most recent OECD data available (OECD 2015), while the United States has increased in recent years in the percentage of the population with at least a high school diploma, it ranks 21 among the OECD nations in student skills as measured by a standard international test. And the higher the level of educational attainment one uses, the worse the United States ranks—10th in having some postsecondary education and 12th in a completed college degree. A major National Academy of Sciences report (2007) highlights these issues. The report emphasizes the role of education in the ability of the United States to compete economically in a world with rapidly expanding educational attainment in many other countries, especially China and India (Phelps 2007). Here I wish to emphasize a different issue—the role of education in changing peoples' lifestyle choices.

I present these data with a small caveat: we can readily observe strong associations between educational attainment and healthy lifestyles. What we cannot know for sure is the ultimate cause. Using smoking as an example, we can be fairly sure that adult smoking habits do not cause lower educational attainment earlier in life. We actually have a decent amount of evidence showing that higher education actually shifts people's lifestyle choices. But there remains a third option—that some unmeasured individual characteristic leads both to more education and improved lifestyle choices (Fuchs 1982). The most obvious factor is differences in the time horizon people hold.[9] Those with a long time horizon will be more apt to invest in more education and also to refrain from poor health habits that lead to poor health outcomes later in life.

My survey of that literature leads me to believe that education is the causative factor. If true, then improving K–12 education will lead people to acquire healthier lifestyles, which will in turn lead to fewer chronic illnesses and lower the rate of growth of future health care spending.

Education and Smoking

First, look at the simple relationship between smoking and educational attainment. No matter how it is measured, higher education is closely linked to lower smoking rates. Figure 2.11 shows the smoking participation rates (smoker vs. nonsmoker) by education.

Perhaps more importantly, Figure 2.11 shows how smoking rates changed after publication of the U.S. surgeon general's report on smoking (U.S. Department of Health, Education, and Welfare 1964). As Fig-

Figure 2.11 Effects of Surgeon General's Report on Smoking, by Educational Attainment

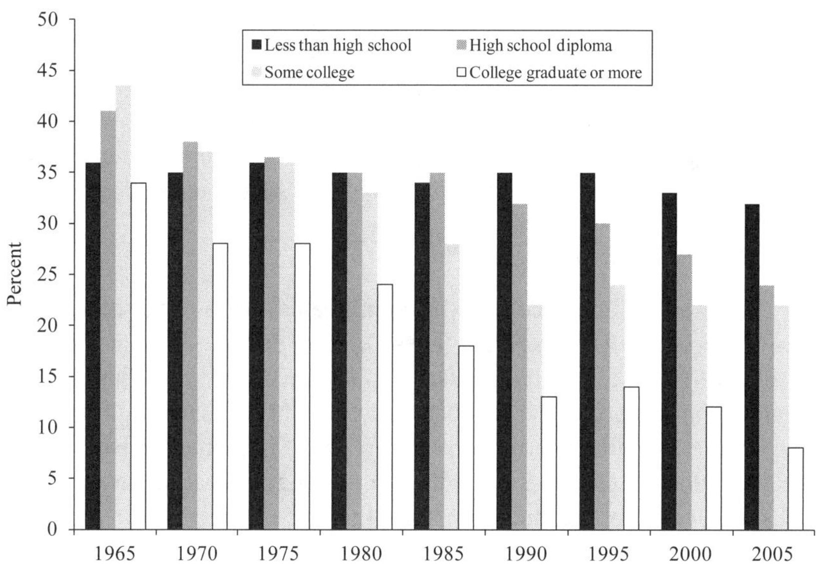

SOURCE: Author's calculations using data from U.S. Public Health Service (various years).

ure 2.7 shows, smoking rates began to plummet in 1965, but the change did not occur equally across educational levels. As Figure 2.11 shows, the rates of those with the least educational attainment changed very little from 1965 onward. Those with the highest educational attainment had the greatest change. Intermediate levels of education show correspondingly intermediate degrees of change in smoking rates.

This is powerful information: higher education, coupled with the new information about the risks of smoking over time, led to far greater reductions in smoking among the most highly educated than for others. The operative mechanism seems to be that those with higher education were able to better understand the new information about smoking risks and incorporate that into their lifestyle choices.

Education and Obesity

We can see the same relationships between obesity (as measured by BMI) and education. Figure 2.12 shows how educational attainment and obesity relate. These data show a steady decline in obesity rates for women (defined as ≥ 25) as educational attainment increases. For men, the data show a slow upward trend in obesity rates until they obtain two years of post–high school education and then strong declines in obesity levels for those completing college and beyond. At all levels of education, obesity rates are higher for men than for women. For women, obesity rates for those who have a college education and above are about half the rates for women with less than a high school education.

Education and Alcohol

As noted before, alcohol is a complicated drug, with some positive and some negative effects. These effects depend on both the type of alcohol and the way it is consumed. Figure 2.13 shows that overall drinking rates increase with educational attainment, seemingly in contrast to the overall patterns seen for smoking and obesity. But within the finer detail of Figure 2.13 we can see that education reduces the rates of alcohol abuse and binge drinking, the types of drinking that lead to poorer health outcomes. Further, when we look at the beverage of choice, higher education is linked to a much stronger preference for wine and less preference for distilled spirits. So, the beverage of choice (wines versus distilled spirits in particular) and the drinking patterns

Figure 2.12 Obesity Rates by Educational Attainment

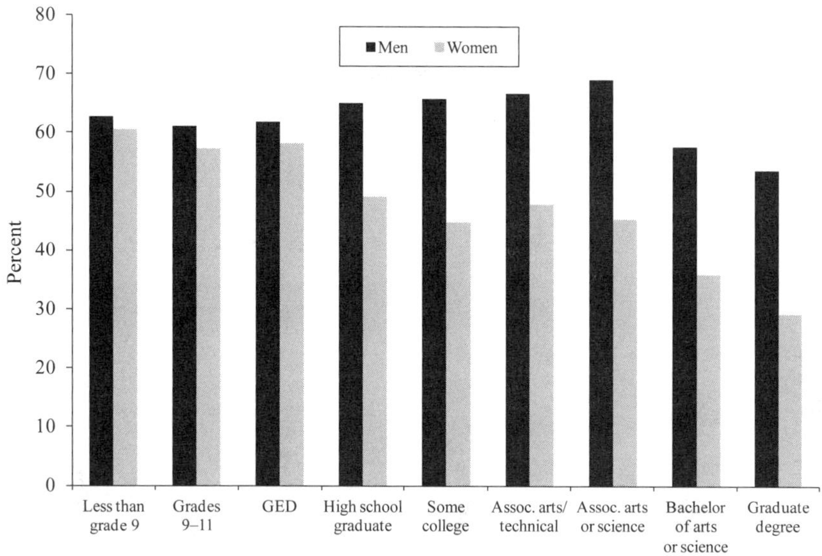

SOURCE: Ogden et al. (2010).

(less binge drinking, less abusive drinking) lead us to the conclusion that people with higher education have in fact made healthier lifestyle choices.

CONCLUSION

Taking aim at our lifestyle choices represents only one of many things we need to do to make our health care system efficient and successful. Many financial incentive problems exist that also need fixing, beginning with the tax subsidy for employer-paid health insurance and ending with major reforms in the structure of Medicare and Medicaid. I address these elsewhere in Phelps (2010). The Affordable Care Act of 2010 fixed a few of the problems described in that book, exacerbated others, and ignored most of the major issues. Moving from that legisla-

Figure 2.13 Alcohol Use, by Educational Attainment

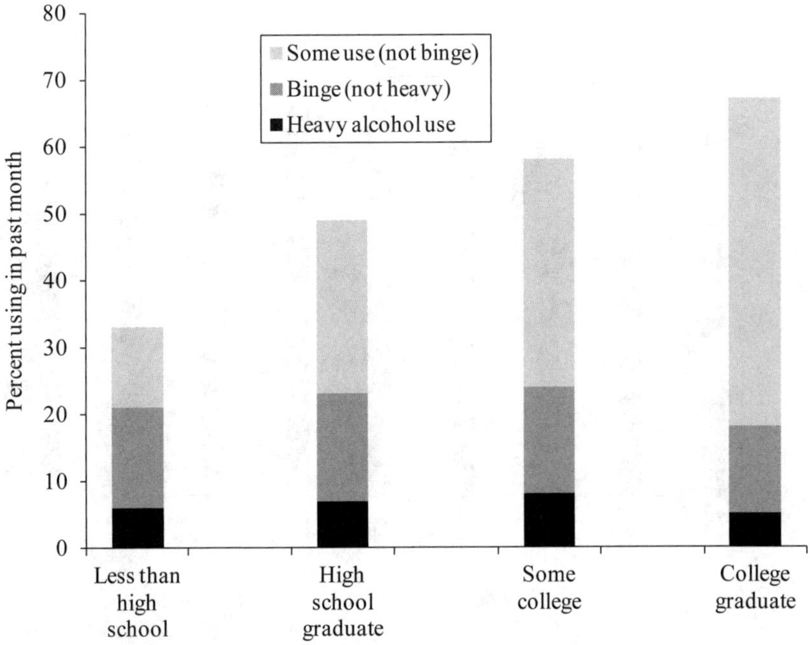

SOURCE: U.S. Department of Health and Human Services (2007).

tion to a system with good protection against financial risk while still maintaining patient and provider incentives for efficient use of health care resources is a subject too broad to cover in this chapter, but it is one that will help define the economic future of the United States.

Notes

1. In economics jargon, the income elasticity is about 1.5, which (strangely to some people) makes health care a "luxury good" by the usual definition—far from a "necessity" or a "human right."
2. Other factors also come into play, including income, cigarette prices, and even wars. As the graph shows, smoking rises dramatically during wartime—that was especially true during World War II, when the Red Cross (and others) gave cigarettes to soldiers.

3. For imperial measurements, use weight in pounds, height in inches, and multiply by 703 to correct for the differences between the measuring systems; thus, BMI = 703 × pounds/(inches × inches).
4. These data come from Calle et al. (1999), a large prospective study of all-cause mortality and BMI. Many other studies exist on this topic; you can find one to give almost any answer you want. For me, the prospective design of this study makes it the gold standard. It began with a fixed group of people and followed their weights and mortality outcomes over time.
5. Heavy drinking is commonly defined as more than 20 drinks per week. Binge drinking has a variety of definitions, the most common being five drinks (four for women) within a two-hour period.
6. The key ingredient appears to be procyanadin (see Corder [2007] for details). For those who prefer to avoid alcohol, other foods with high levels of procyanadin include chocolate, cranberry juice, pomegranates, and certain types of apples. It seems that an apple a day may in fact keep the doctor away.
7. In computerese, we have "garbage in, garbage out." Here we have "fat in, fat out."
8. For example, to have a BMI of 40, a person measuring 5'6" would have to weigh at least 247 pounds, and a person 6'0" would have to weigh at least 294 pounds.
9. Economists examine this issue by looking at the internal discount rate, the rate at which things that occur in the future are valued less. Think about savings behavior (as a simple investment) and the interest rate banks will pay you. If they pay 1 percent above inflation, you are not likely to save much, but if they pay 10 percent above inflation, you will save much more. Time discounting works similarly (but in the opposite direction)—those with a high discount rate save (or invest) less for the future.

References

Calle, Eugenia E., Michael J. Thun, Jennifer M. Petrelli, Carmen Rodriguez, and Clark W. Heath, Jr. 1999. "Body-Mass Index and Mortality in a Prospective Cohort of U.S. Adults." *New England Journal of Medicine* 341: 1097–1105.

Corder, Roger. 2007. *The Red Wine Diet*. New York: The Penguin Group.

Estruch, Ramón, Emilio Ros, Jordi Salas-Salvadó, Maria-Isabel Covas, Dolores Corella, Fernando Arós, Enrique Gómez-Gracia, Valentina Ruiz-Gutiérrez, Miquel Fiol, José Lapetra, Rosa Maria Lamuela-Raventos, Lluís Serra-Majem, Xavier Pintó, Josep Basora, Miguel Angel Muñoz, José V. Sorlí, José Alfredo Martínez, and Miguel Angel Martínez-González. 2013. "Primary Prevention of Cardiovascular Disease with a Mediterranean Diet." *New England Journal of Medicine* 368: 1279–1290.

Finkelstein, Eric A., Justin G. Trogdon, Joel W. Cohen, and William Dietz. 2009. "Annual Medical Spending Attributable to Obesity: Payer-and-Service-Specific Estimates." *Health Affairs* 28(5): w822–w831.

Fuchs, Victor R. 1982. "Time Preference and Health: An Exploratory Study." In *Economic Aspects of Health*, Victor R. Fuchs, ed. Chicago: University of Chicago Press, pp. 93–120.

Grønbaek, Morten, Ulrik Becker, Ditte Johansen, Adam Gottschau, Peter Schnohr, Hans Ole Hein, Gorm Jensen, and Thorkild I.A. Sørensen. 2000. "Type of Alcohol Consumed and Mortality from All Causes, Coronary Heart Disease, and Cancer." *Annals of Internal Medicine* 133(6): 411–419.

Hughes, John R., and Anthony Liguori. 2000. "A Critical View of Past NIH Research Funding on Tobacco and Nicotine." *Nicotine Tobacco Research* 2(2): 117–120.

Kolonel L. N., M. W. Hinds, and J. H. Hankin. 1980. "Cancer Patterns among Migrant and Native-Born Japanese in Hawaii in Relation to Smoking, Drinking, and Dietary Habits." In *Genetic and Environmental Factors in Experimental and Human Cancer*, Harry Victor Gelboin and Takamatsu no Miya Hi Gan Kenkyū Kikin, eds. Tokyo: Sci. Soc. Press, pp. 327–340.

Manning,William G., Emmett B. Keeler, Joseph P. Newhouse, Elizabeth M. Sloss, and Jeffrey Wasserman. 1989. "The Taxes of Sin: Do Smokers and Drinkers Pay Their Way?" *Journal of the American Medical Association* 261(11): 1604–1609.

McGinnis, J. Michael, and William H. Foege. 1993. "Actual Causes of Death in the United States." *Journal of the American Medical Association* 270(18): 2207–2212.

Mokdad, Ali H., James S. Marks, Donna F. Stroup, and Julie L. Gerberding. 2004. "Actual Causes of Death in the United States, 2000." *Journal of the American Medical Association* 291(10): 1238–1245.

National Academy of Sciences. 2007. *Rising above the Gathering Storm: Energizing and Employing America for a Brighter Economic Future*. Washington, DC: National Academies Press. Committee on Prospering in the Global Economy of the 21st Century: An Agenda for American Science and Technology; Committee on Science, Engineering, and Public Policy; Institute of Medicine; Policy and Global Affairs; National Academy of Sciences; National Academy of Engineering.

Ogden, Cynthia L., Molly M. Lamb, Margaret D. Carroll, and Katherine M. Flegal. 2010. "Obesity and Socioeconomic Status in Adults: United States, 2005–2008." NCHS Data Brief No. 50. Washington, DC: U.S. Department of Health and Human Services, National Center for Health Statistics.

Organisation for Economic Co-operation and Development (OECD). 2015. *Education at a Glance, 2014*. Paris: OECD Indicators. DOI: http://dx.doi.org/10.1787/eag-2014-en (accessed September 8, 2015).

Phelps, Charles E. 2007. "Globalization of Higher Education." *Advancing Higher Education*. New York: TIAA-CREF Institute. https://www

.tiaainstitute.org/public/pdf/institute/research/advancing_higher_education/inst_advancing_higher_ed_phelps_112707.pdf (accessed September 8, 2015).

———. 2010. *Eight Questions You Should Ask about Our Health Care System (Even If the Answers Make You Sick)*. Stanford, CA: Hoover Institution Press.

Rand, Ayn. 1943. *The Fountainhead*. Indianapolis: Bobbs-Merrill Company.

Stewart, Susan T., David M. Cutler, and Allison B. Rosen. 2009. "Forecasting the Effects of Obesity and Smoking on U.S. Life Expectancy." *New England Journal of Medicine* 361(23): 2252–2260.

Tanabe, Marianne K.G. N.d. "Health and Health Care of Japanese-American Elders." Honolulu: John A. Burns School of Medicine, University of Hawaii. http://web.stanford.edu/group/ethnoger/japanese.html (accessed January 11, 2016).

U.S. Department of Health, Education, and Welfare. 1964. *Smoking and Health: Report of the Advisory Committee to the Surgeon General of the Public Health Service*. Public Health Service Publication No. 1103. Washington, DC: U.S. Department of Health, Education, and Welfare.

U.S. Department of Health and Human Services. 2007. "2007 National Survey on Drug Use and Health." Washington, DC: Substance Abuse and Mental Health Services Administration, Center for Behavioral Health Statistics and Quality.

Warner, K. E. 1989. "Effects of the Antismoking Campaign: An Update." *American Journal of Public Health* 79(2): 144–151.

Wunsch, Hannah, Walter T. Linde-Zwirble, David A. Harrison, Amber E. Barnato, Kathryn M. Rowan, and Derek C. Angus. 2009. "Use of Intensive Care Services during Terminal Hospitalizations in England and the United States." *American Journal of Respiratory and Critical Care Medicine* 180: 875–880.

3
Do Medical Care and Self-Care Compete or Complement in Health Production?

Donald J. Meyer
Western Michigan University

Modern medical care is a major determinant of one's health. Many of us obtain better health from visiting a doctor when we are sick and, when necessary, seeking diagnostic laboratory and imaging tests, medicine, hospital care, and outpatient surgery. Our own self-care is equally important for maintaining good health, as are preventative measures we take that either reduce the probability of sickness, illness, or accident or lower the severity of the health event. Dow, Philipson, and Sala-I-Martin (1999) cite the importance of both of these health inputs: "Resources devoted to extending life may be interpreted not only as medical care (e.g., hospital and physician services), but also as expenditures on dietary needs, home care, physical exercise, or even time transfers from children or spouses at old age" (p. 1360). The question of interest for this chapter is, do people use these two factor types more in conjunction with each other, or do they generally use one in place of the other?

One argument is that these two inputs are best used together—that is, they are complementary. Becker (2007) examines health as a type of human capital and looks at how it fits in with other forms of human capital. To do this, he uses a survivor risk model of expected utility. The uncertainty in the model refers to how long one lives or survives from one period to the next. This survivorship probability depends on the level of various health inputs, health shock events, and other factors. He notes that the health field is full of complementarities such as that between various diseases or health conditions. An increase in the probability of surviving one disease (due to one form of treatment) enhances or raises the additional benefit from spending on other treatments to help survive other diseases. Becker also notes similar complementarities between health and education, between age levels, and between health and the discount rate.

A second argument is that these two inputs are used in competition with one another—that is, we tend to substitute one input for the other. Consider someone who has been diagnosed with a high blood pressure condition. This condition may be treated with better lifestyle habits, such as losing weight, increasing regular exercise, and limiting sodium intake, or with various types of prescribed blood pressure medications and pills. If some medications are newly taken, do you respond by exercising less and eating more salt in your diet since the medicine is now taking care of the condition? Or, consider someone who previously had no health care or health insurance and now obtains it as a part of the Affordable Care Act. Does this person rely more on the modern medical care system to take care of his health needs and health level determination and thus worry less about maintaining a healthy lifestyle?

The United States spends more per capita on health care than any other country. We have some of the most advanced health care technologies in the world. However, we have higher infant mortality rates and a lower life expectancy rate than many other countries (Phelps 2010, pp. 6–7). Additionally, we have one of the highest obesity rates in the world, as well as low levels of exercise. How much are our lifestyle choices linked to a substitution effect of experiencing newer and better modern medical care? Can we take measures to reduce this offset effect on health levels as new technological advances emerge?

The rest of the chapter is organized as follows. In the next section, I provide background information about good health modeling and present some traditional ideas about input substitution and complementarity. The third section argues the need to view demand and production of health in a model of uncertainty. This uncertainty model framework then gets applied to health with some important differences noted from the basic model. I then examine the notion of modern care and self-care being substitutes versus complements in this context. The section after that examines three papers that contribute to this discussion, and the final section offers concluding remarks.

BACKGROUND INFORMATION

As consumers, we often do not think regularly about production functions and their related concepts. I envision here a health production function, $H = f$(medical care, self-care, education, family genes, environment), for which the first two factors receive the focus or attention in this chapter. We are more familiar, perhaps, with our preferences and demand for the various goods and services that are in our utility functions. A common health formulation for utility is the function $U = U(H, Z)$, where utility depends on one's health level, H, and the amount consumed of a composite or a home-produced good Z. Health is an interesting and challenging good to model in this way. As Grossman (1972) notes in his seminal article, health is part consumption good (we enjoy good health), part input into the production or purchase of good Z, and part capital stock or durable good. H is a stock for which the level increases through investment and deteriorates over time from depreciation.

I do not go into the determination of selecting an optimal level of H (and Z) to maximize utility in this chapter, but I do assume that the consumer solves this maximization problem. A unique and important feature about H is that it cannot be purchased in the marketplace; that is, we cannot specialize in producing Z and then trade some of it for H. Whatever H level we wish to consume must also be produced. This validates the importance of focusing on health production and the emphasis on the two inputs noted in the chapter and the relationship that exists between them.

For a neoclassical, nonstochastic production function, there are two traditional ways to classify two factors or inputs as substitutes, complements, or neither. One definition is to look at what happens to the marginal productivity of factor 2 when the decision maker uses a greater level of input 1. Two factors are complements when an increase in factor 1 enhances the marginal productivity of factor 2. Two factors are substitutes when an increase in factor 1 reduces the marginal product of factor 2. Two factors are neither (or neutral) when the marginal productivity of factor 2 has no relation to the level of input 1. So, ditch diggers and shovels would be complements if the workers became more productive moving dirt with a shovel than without. Grocery store checkers and self-scanning devices may be substitutes if the productivity of checkers falls as self-scanning devices become available for grocery checkout.

A second definition involves what happens to the demand for factor 2 if the price of factor 1 were to increase. Two inputs are complements when an increase in the price of factor 1 leads to a reduction in demand for factor 2. Two factors are substitutes if an increase in the price of factor 1 leads to an increase in demand for factor 2. So, looking at the same two examples, ditch diggers and shovels are classified as complements because an increase in the price of ditch diggers would reduce the demand for shovels. Grocery store checkers and self-scanners are classified as substitutes because an increase in the wage of checkers would increase the demand for self-scanning devices.

Now let's apply these definitions to health and self-care. If your employer provides you with a subsidized health club and personal trainer membership, then complementarity suggests that your health insurance and medical care become more effective. Or, if you obtain medical care through the Affordable Care Act, the substitution effect suggests you would rely more on medical care and reduce your effort with self-care. While this traditional pair of definitions is useful and somewhat helpful in thinking about how medical care and self-care are related, I argue next that we need to consider health production and consumption in a context of uncertainty and model it as such. That is, random health events, health losses, or disease outbreak must be considered to affect *H* along with the first two inputs and other factors already considered.

UNCERTAINTY CONSIDERATIONS AND CONTEXT

The process of attempting to attain one's desired health stock is subject to much randomness and uncertainty. Health losses are possible, owing to contracting any one of a number of debilitating diseases, or suffering relapses during the recovery process. Automobile or other types of accidents can drastically alter one's health status in a matter of moments. How one will respond to prescribed medical treatment is never certain. Dardanoni and Wagstaff (1990) note these sources of health uncertainty and also the presence of imperfect information regarding assessment of either the effectiveness of medical care or of one's health level itself. Health decision making is subject to random influences, and determination of possible outcomes and the associated probabilities is certainly a subjective evaluation process. It is essential that the relation between modern health treatment and self-care be examined within the context of this uncertain environment.

As I address some of the basics for decision making under uncertainty, I will highlight the ideas of risk and risk aversion, and also the idea of turning to organized insurance markets as a way to shift risk to a third party. I then examine self-care, where I refer to the ideas of self-protection and self-insurance. I first review this material in general and then apply it to our specific health setting, incorporating some of the unique features of health. I will then summarize what is predicted or known regarding the substitution or complementary nature of medical care and self-care.

Consider the simple expected utility, additive formulation for a risky setting: $W_f = W_0 + V - L$, where W_f is final wealth, W_0 is nonrandom initial wealth, V is the value of a risky asset, and L is random loss associated with V. V could be one's house, automobile, life or earning potential, or one's health stock. V is subject to losses, L, of uncertain magnitude. Wealth at the end of the period reflects whatever losses regarding L are incurred. It is generally assumed that one can list all possible outcomes for L and the associated probabilities for all the outcomes. For simplicity, it has often assumed that losses follow a Bernoulli distribution; that is, have loss L_1 with probability p or no loss with probability $1-p$.

How does one view facing this uncertain value for V? Risk aversion is the norm, where risk aversion means a distaste or disutility for the randomness one is facing. A risk-averse person is generally willing to pay for a reduction in risk; this leads to a basic trade-off between risk and return or income. Market insurance is a common way to shift risk to an outside agent for a fee or payment.

The basic insurance contract has two main features: 1) the indemnity function, which describes what the insurance company will pay the policy holder for various levels of L; and 2) the insurance payment or premium. The premium paid directly depends not on the value of L but on the expected value of L. Common forms for insurance policies are deductible and coinsurance. The premium will depend on the deductible or copay rate that is selected by the policy holder. Deductible insurance has the desirable feature of offering greater coverage for high-loss values, but it offers less coverage when losses are small and easier to be covered by the individual.

Insurance policies can offer larger or smaller levels of coverage. Premiums reflect the level of protection that is selected in the policy. The premium paid for a policy is generally equal to or larger than the expected loss for *L*. A premium equal to the expected loss is said to be "actuarially fair"—that is, the insurance company will break even on average for such policies. The amount collected in premiums will just cover what is paid out for losses on average. Premiums are often higher than this break-even level to cover overhead and related costs of providing service. The fundamental theorem of insurance coverage states that if offered insurance at an actuarially fair rate, all risk-averse persons will choose full or 100 percent coverage.

Self-care measures can be taken in conjunction with market insurance or when formal insurance is not available in the marketplace. Self-insurance refers to undertaking an expenditure that lowers the size of *L*, and self-protection refers to undertaking an expenditure to lower the probability of incurring a given loss. As Ehrlich and Becker (1972) note, some self-care choices fall in the self-insurance category, some are of the self-protection variety, and some have aspects of both types. Common examples of self-insurance are installing fire sprinklers to guard against fire damage, using sturdier building materials in earthquake- and hurricane-prone areas, and installing a tracking device in a car to make recovery easier when stolen. Self-protection measures include installing home security protection to help keep burglars out, efforts to reduce the probability of a terrorist attack, or using a steering wheel locking device to reduce the chance of theft. Ehrlich and Becker suggest that a talented lawyer serves to reduce both the chance of a criminal conviction and possibly the severity of the sentencing.

Ehrlich and Becker (1972) is a highly cited article and is foundational in the self-care literature. The authors look at the market insurance option as a means of risk reduction along with the ideas of self-insurance and self-protection. They suggest that when addressing the need to limit one's risk position, one should look at all three of these together, as each serves to deal with loss reduction or loss likelihood in one fashion or another. They also note that both market insurance and self-insurance work to shift income toward the loss state and hence tend to be substitutes for each other.

Self-protection, on the other hand, reduces income in both the loss and no-loss state by the cost of the activity, offering the benefit of reducing the probability of the negative event. It is considerably more complex in its effect on the risk problem and offers less clear-cut results or findings. Ehrlich and Becker (1972) find that self-protection and market insurance tend to be complementary in nature rather than substitutes, with the strength of the complementarity depending on market conditions. Many others have followed up this initial work with a focus on self-protection, owing to its more challenging nature and complexity.

Dionne and Eeckhoudt (1985) explore the relationship between increasing risk aversion and self-insurance and self-protection. The first idea is expected: as people become more risk averse, their level of self-insurance increases. However, the authors find that self-protection is not monotonically related to the level of risk aversion. They look for conditions that would allow more precise findings about how increased risk aversion and self-protection are related, but few clean and intuitive results were able to be reached. They did look at the relation for two specific utility preferences: a quadratic utility maximizer and a logarithmic utility function. For two logarithmic expected utility maximizers with different levels of risk aversion, they find that the more risk-averse person actually chose less self-protection.

Briys and Schlesinger (1990) build on these two papers and look further at risk aversion and self-protection and self-insurance. They broaden the known results for self-insurance by showing that under state-dependent utility and in the presence of background risk, self-insurance and risk aversion continue to be directly related. The authors make the revealing observation that self-protection can be broken down into a combination of a mean-preserving spread and a mean-preserving contraction. The spread occurs at a lower level of the decision maker's income, and the contraction takes place at a higher income level.

Eeckhoudt and Gollier (2005) apply a different uncertainty concept, prudence, to the analysis of self-protection. Prudence, which exists when the third derivative of the utility function is positive, differentiates between the risk occurring in the upper versus lower end of the income distribution. The authors show that prudence, as well as the probability of the loss being closer to unity versus closer to zero, is crucial in self-protection determination. Meyer and Meyer (2011) further clarify with additional analysis the role that prudence plays for self-protection. Their findings hinge on the size of the risk increase (in the lower end of income distribution) versus the size of the risk decrease (in the upper end of income distribution). Meyer and Meyer's results use a risk technique introduced by Diamond and Sitglitz (1974), which considerably simplifies the analysis and allows for generalization. For example, the loss distribution was allowed to be more general and not required to follow the often-assumed Bernoulli distribution.

Finally, Snow (2011) looks at self-protection and self-insurance from a nonexpected utility framework. He integrates the concept of ambiguity and ambiguity aversion to his analysis of self-care. Ambiguity exists when there is uncertainty about the probability of the loss occurring. In the expected utility model, the probabilities concerning losses are assumed to be known with certainty. He shows that optimal levels of self-protection and self-insurance are higher in the presence of ambiguity (than with none) or when people are more ambiguity averse. A significant difference between Snow's and much of the prior results is that his findings are similar for both self-protection and self-insurance, rather than differing considerably in the literature that uses expected utility formulation.

So what does decision making under uncertainty—in particular, market insurance, self-insurance, and self-protection—have to do with the relationship between modern medical care and self-care in the health setting? The answer lies in considering how these concepts apply to the analysis of making decisions under health uncertainty. The particular manner in which health markets function turns out to be critical in this discussion. First, it is important to recognize the close link between health insurance and modern medical care. The typical health insurance policy covers a large number of medical health care items and procedures. Health insurance is essentially prepaid medical care, as it covers most of your medical expenses. Unlike other forms of insurance, you do not receive monetary payment from the insurance company based on the health loss that you have experienced. Instead, you seek medical treatment for your health issue, and then insurance pays much of these medical bills. Self-care undertakings and efforts are typically not covered by one's health insurance. Self-protection and self-insurance strategies undertaken on an individual level are paid for by the individual.

Approximately 50 percent of U.S. residents receive health insurance and medical care through their employers. The roots for this program go back to the 1940s, when firms, which were facing both wage controls and a shortage of workers in World War II, started offering health insurance as a nontaxable employee benefit. The idea was positively received by workers and has become integrated as part of our national health care system. Even so, a sizable percentage of Americans have had to do without health insurance. The Affordable Care Act is working to reduce this number, as those who previously had no health insurance are able to obtain it through their state health exchange system or through the Medicaid expansions.

As an example of a typical health insurance policy and the medical care that is covered, I will examine the policy that I have at Western Michigan University. Blue Cross Blue Shield of Michigan provides a Preferred Provider Organization policy for university employees. This type of policy allows one to seek medical care from any provider desired but offers a financial incentive to seek treatment from a provider who is part of the network or system. My policy covers most types of medical care, including primary or specialist care visits, diagnostic or imaging tests, prescription drugs, outpatient center and surgeon services, emergency and urgent care treatment, and hospital care. The policy carefully gives all the deductibles and copays that must be paid in the different situations. Some medical treatments, such as acupuncture, cosmetic surgery, and weight loss programs, are not covered by the policy.

Several features of health insurance work to reinforce this close tie between insurance and medical care. First, health insurance typically covers routine medical care, such as a doctor's visit or an antibiotics prescription. Most other forms of insurance are more of a "catastrophic coverage" nature only and do not cover the routine expenditures. Second, the monetary indemnity payment received from non-health types of insurance policies is based on the loss that is experienced regarding your risky asset. Money payment is sent directly to the person who experiences roof hail damage, based on an independent assessment of the damage. For health insurance, no such money payment is received; rather, the health care provider receives payment for health services rendered in treating the health condition. Lastly, the insurance relation, in reality, is between the insurance company and the health care provider—in most loss instances the patient has little direct involvement in the exchange. All of these serve to strengthen the connection between health insurance and modern medical care.

Second, self-care in the health setting—self-protection and self-insurance—is reflected mainly in wise lifestyle choices that involve eating, exercise, tobacco and alcohol usage, and stress management. Sticking to a healthy diet and controlling one's weight reduces the chances of coronary disease due to high blood pressure or of developing type II diabetes. By exercising and keeping fit, one lowers the chances of developing any number of negative health issues and also enhances recovery when illness develops or surgery is required. Overuse of alcohol or tobacco products has negative effects on your health, and such products should be eliminated or used in moderation. Wise lifestyle choices can both reduce the likelihood of a bad health event and reduce the loss if such an event does occur.

The primary question of interest for this chapter is whether medical care and lifestyle choices (self-care) are more of a complementary or substitution type of relationship. The purpose of this section has been to prove that this must be examined within a risk and uncertainty context using the related concepts of market insurance, self-protection, and self-insurance. This leads to a much richer and more relevant definition of substitutes and complements in production of health than the simple neoclassical production formulation discussed earlier.

So, where do I stand on this question? It remains an empirical issue—both the substitution and complementarity effects are legitimate and are possible in every situation; the size of each effect will depend on the particular setting one is in and in how medical or self-care is being measured. Both types of care are broad concepts, there is not likely to be just a single relationship between them. Substitution between medical care and self-care is a strong force and is more likely to be readily apparent. Complementarity is more subtle and will likely be more difficult to observe, and its statistical significance is less clear. As Dow, Philipson, and Sala-I-Martin (1999) note, "Although complementarity induced by competing risks applies very generally, the important question for evaluating public health programs is whether its empirical magnitude is significant" (p. 1359).

A REVIEW OF THREE EMPIRICAL PAPERS

In this section I review three papers that focus on the relationship between some aspect of the modern medical care system together with different features of self-care. The first paper looks at implementation in developing countries of the Expanded Programme on Immunization (EPI) of the United Nations. The expected immunization of children against the six deadliest childhood diseases caused mothers to take better care of their children in general, which supports the complementarity effect. The next paper examines the effect Medicare had on the health behaviors of new Medicare enrollees in the United States. The authors find evidence of ex ante moral hazard, or the substitution effect of those receiving Medicare taking less good care of their health. The final paper discusses the effect that statin drugs, which are very successful in treating high cholesterol and heart disease, have on the lifestyle choices of those using the statins. Strong evidence for substitution is noted, as people may feel able to get away with a less healthy lifestyle given they have this "get out of jail free card." Some positive, though more uneven, evidence of significant complementarity was also found.

Dow, Philipson, and Sala-I-Martin (1999) examine household data for four African countries—Malawi, Tanzania, Zambia, and Zimbabwe—for children who are expected to receive vaccinations for measles, neonatal tetanus, polio, whooping cough, diphtheria, and tuberculosis. The authors hypothesize that women will seek better nutrition and other health inputs when they believe that their children will be inoculated against these potentially fatal childhood diseases. The researchers use birth weight as the indicator of maternal care.

Using data on the children, ordinary least squares estimates are first calculated, followed by estimates from present family fixed effects and lagged instrumental fixed effects models, owing to concern for possible unobserved heterogeneity in the data. Other safeguards and robustness checks are implemented as well. The authors consistently find complementarity between the care taken by mothers and the expected vaccinations against the diseases.

Dow, Philipson, and Sala-I-Martin (1999) argue for the significance of these complementarity effects in health mortalities programs, such as the EPI in developing countries. Treatment for one set of diseases has positive spillover effects on the mortality rates of other health issues. If one were to consider the marginal benefit and marginal costs of the treatment or programs in isolation from each other, then erroneous conclusions would be reached regarding implementation levels of these treatments. For this particular health setting or environment, it seems that complementarity is evident, real, and sizable, and it needs to be incorporated into the health analysis.

Dave and Kaestner (2009) find strong evidence of substitution away from healthy lifestyle choice in response to new availability and lower costs of medical provisions from Medicare. They identify direct or ex ante moral hazard effect in conjunction with a secondary indirect effect. This so-called doctor effect is because increased physician contact from Medicare alters information concerning the benefits of self-care leading to better lifestyle choices. Dave and Kaestner estimate both of these countervailing effects and in general find significance for both.

The authors look at three lifestyle choice behaviors separately for both males and females—exercise, smoking, and alcohol use. Results for men are largely statistically significant and show that Medicare led to a worsening of healthy lifestyle choices. For the sample of males the authors find a decrease in the probability of vigorous physical exercise, higher prevalence of daily smoking along with increased cigarette consumption, and an increase in probable alcohol use, including daily. The same estimates for women are generally statistically insignificant, although Medicare is generally associated with a worsening of lifestyle choices.

Kaestner, Darden, and Lakdawalla (2014) search for both substitution and complementarity effects on lifestyle choice variables due to statin drug use. Statins have been shown to significantly reduce cardiovascular disease and health complications due to high cholesterol. One may be tempted to forgo costly lifestyle choices known to combat high cholesterol and related issues while on a statin prescription. The complementarity effect, on the other hand, suggests that if statin use decreases the problems related to heart disease, one has an increased incentive to make healthier choices that reduce the mortality from other diseases.

The substitution effect is seen by an increase in the body mass index and the likelihood of being obese, an increase in moderate alcohol use by men, and a decrease in exercise rates for women. The authors also find some evidence of complementarity, however, in the form of higher physical activity for males and greater use of preventative medicines, such as blood pressure medication and aspirin, for both genders.

Furthermore, Kaestner, Darden, and Lakdawalla (2014) write, "There is a general concern that statin use may adversely affect health behaviors that substitute for pharmaceutical treatment of hyperlipidemia. If there is substitution of statins for a healthy lifestyle, then the efficacy of statin use may be compromised and statin use may result in a greater incidence of disease that is unrelated to cholesterol, but associated with a healthy lifestyle (diet and exercise)" (p. 162).

CONCLUDING THOUGHTS

There is a need for additional empirical work that looks for the possible presence and magnitude of both the substitution and complementarity effects as we continue to gather evidence and sort out the connection between medical care and self-care. Abrokwah, Callison, and Meyer (2015) examine the rollout of nationalized health care in Ghana in 2004. Tentatively, after the rollout they not only find evidence for the substitution toward medical care away from alternative or traditional care but also observe complementarity between some specific forms of alternative or traditional care and medical care.

Furthermore, as already noted, complementarities create spillover effects due to competing risks in the survival model. As Dow, Philipson, and Sala-I-Martin (1999) suggest, the marginal benefit of investing in lowering the mortality rate for one disease can increase as the survival rates for other diseases or health conditions increase. The decision maker needs to recognize the private benefit from this positive externality when selecting his or her optimal mix of health inputs. Incorporating this on an individual basis will strengthen health as a positive externality for overall society as well. Every one of us benefits as a larger percentage of people seek and reach good health status. On the flip side, the negative externalities resulting from obesity, excessive spending in the last few months of life, and poor lifestyle can affect everyone, too.

To more fully benefit from these positive spillovers, measures could be taken that support or subsidize the complementarity between inputs and that limit excessive substitution between the inputs. For example, through various forms of media or advertising, people can be encouraged to prepare healthy meals or to engage in exercise. Visually portraying a group of bicyclists or runners laughing and having a good time or showing a family having quality time preparing and eating a meal together can strengthen the positive consumption feature that good health provides. This would not only increase health levels of individuals, but on a larger scale could also help reduce our excessive health spending and increase our national health performance measures.

References

Abrokwah, Stephen O., K. Callison, and Donald Meyer. 2015. "The Relationship between Modern and Traditional Care in Developing Countries." Unpublished paper, Western Michigan University, Kalamazoo, MI.

Becker, Gary S. 2007. "Health as Human Capital: Synthesis and Extensions." *Oxford Economic Papers* 59(3): 379–410.

Briys, Eric, and Harris Schlesinger. 1990. "Risk Aversion and the Propensities for Self-Insurance and Self-Protection." *Southern Economic Journal* 57(2): 458–467.

Dardanoni, Valentino, and Adam Wagstaff. 1990. "Uncertainty and the Demand for Medical Care." *Journal of Health Economics* 9(1): 23–38.

Dave, Dharal, and Robert Kaestner. 2009. "Health Insurance and Ex Ante Moral Hazard: Evidence from Medicare." *International Journal of Health Care Finance and Economics* 9(4): 367–390.

Diamond, Peter A., and Joseph E. Stiglitz. 1974. "Increases in Risk and in Risk Aversion." *Journal of Economic Theory* 8(3): 337–360.

Dionne, Georges, and Louis Eeckhoudt. 1985. "Self-Insurance, Self-Protection, and Increased Risk Aversion." *Economics Letters* 17(1-2): 39–42.

Dow, William H., Tomas J. Philipson, and Xavier Sala-I-Martin. 1999. "Longevity Complementarities under Competing Risks." *American Economic Review* 89(5): 1358–1371.

Eeckhoudt, Louis, and Christian Gollier. 2005. "The Impact of Prudence on Optimal Prevention." *Economic Theory* 26(4): 989–994.

Ehrlich, Isaac, and Gary S. Becker. 1972. "Market Insurance, Self-Insurance and Self-Protection." *Journal of Political Economy* 80(4): 623–648.

Grossman, Michael. 1972. "On the Concept of Health Capital and the Demand for Health." *Journal of Political Economy* 80(2): 223–255.

Kaestner, Robert, Michael Darden, and Darius Lakdawalla. 2014. "Are Investments in Disease Prevention Complements? The Case of Statins and Health Behaviors." *Journal of Health Economics* 36: 151–163.

Meyer, Donald, and Jack Meyer. 2011. "A Diamond-Stiglitz Approach to the Demand for Self-Protection." *Journal of Risk and Uncertainty* 42(1): 45–60.

Phelps, Charles E. 2010. *Eight Questions You Should Ask about Our Health Care System (Even If the Answers Make You Sick)*. Stanford, CA: Hoover Institution Press.

Snow, Arthur. 2011. "Ambiguity Aversion and the Propensities for Self-Insurance and Self-Protection." *Journal of Risk and Uncertainty* 42(1): 27–43.

4
Payment Reform and "Bending the Curve"

John H. Goddeeris
Michigan State University

> *"It's important for us to bend the cost curve . . . because the system we have right now is unsustainable . . ."*
> —President Barack Obama, *Washington Post*, July 22, 2009

WHAT CURVE AND WHY BEND IT?

The need to "bend the curve" is a constant refrain in discussions of health care policy. President Obama emphasized it as one of his two major objectives in promoting health care reform, the other being to greatly increase the number of insured. Numerous academic studies, newspaper articles, and blog posts have debated whether the Affordable Care Act (ACA) will succeed in bending the curve and discussed additional steps that could help. Everyone seems to agree that bending the curve is something we must do.

So, what is this curve that everyone wants to bend? Those who use the expression are not always explicit about what they mean, but one possibility is the curve showing the time trend of the share of gross domestic product (GDP) devoted to health care, as in Figure 4.1. This curve is not exactly smooth, especially over the last two decades, but the long-term trend is upward, with national health expenditures rising from 5.2 percent of GDP in 1960 to 17.5 percent in 2014. Clearly there is some indication that this curve has already been bent, as the share of GDP has been essentially flat since 2009. Nonetheless, government forecasters still expect the share to rise to 19.6 percent by 2024 (Keehan et al. 2015).

Figure 4.1 Health Care as a Percent of GDP (through 2014)

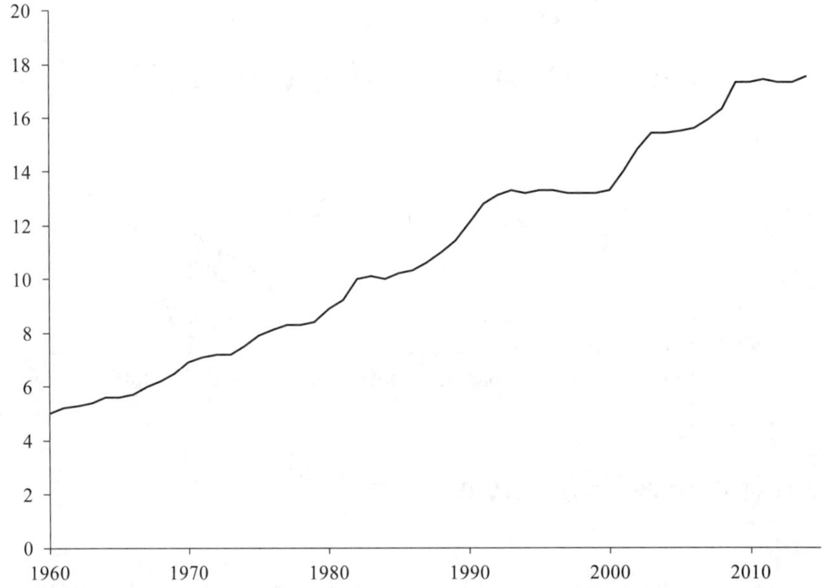

It may seem obvious that we should want to see a permanent plateau in the curve in Figure 4.1, but not everyone would agree. Economists Robert Hall and Charles Jones (2007) have argued that as our standard of living improves (they expect, perhaps optimistically, a return to more traditional levels of economic growth), it is perfectly natural that we would devote a larger share of our resources to longer lives and better health. According to their models, 30 percent of GDP devoted to health by 2050 may be just what we want.

Given the nature of our political system, the curve that may need to be bent more urgently concerns the part of health care spending financed through government. Although the United States arguably has the lowest level of government involvement in its health care system among advanced countries, our government's share of total health spending was already at 47 percent in 2013.

The Congressional Budget Office (CBO) has for a number of years warned about the challenge that health care spending growth poses for the federal government. Figure 4.2 shows recent trends and projections as of June 2015 of federal spending (excluding interest on the debt) separated into components, assuming current law remains in place (CBO 2015). While the recent slowdown in the growth of health spending has had a favorable impact on the budget, the figure shows that major health programs are still projected to claim a larger share of GDP over time, growing at a faster rate than Social Security. The projected decline relative to the economy of other noninterest spending, which includes national defense, may also prove difficult to accomplish.

Furthermore, over the long run, while population aging and the expansion of coverage under health care reform are also important factors, much of the growth of federal health care spending is about increases in spending on a per beneficiary basis, what the CBO calls "excess cost growth." Projecting out to the year 2040, the CBO attributes 45 percent of the growth of major health programs relative to GDP to excess cost growth (CBO 2015, p. 25).[1]

One response to these projections, in line with the Hall and Jones (2007) findings, is that if they prove to be correct we must simply find

Figure 4.2 Trends in Components of Federal Spending as a Percent of GDP

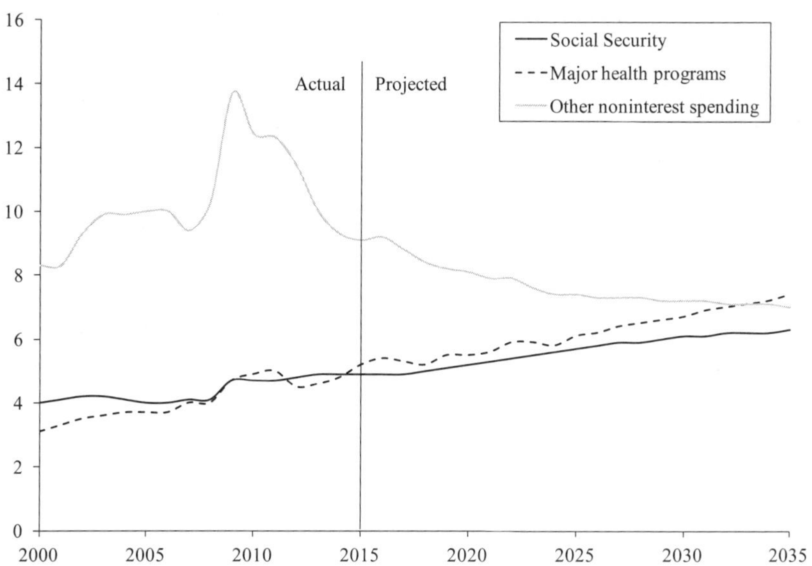

the necessary revenue, because we place a high and increasing value on the improvements in health made possible by rising health spending. Such a response seems to underplay the political difficulties of significantly increasing the share of GDP taken in taxes, as well as the competing pressures to increase other forms of spending, such as on defense, homeland security, education, and infrastructure.

In addition, there is a widely shared view that we are not getting enough from the resources we currently devote to health care—that we ought to be able to slow the growth of health spending without significant sacrifice. The United States spends far and away the largest share of GDP on health care of any country, yet it lags behind other advanced countries in such health indicators as life expectancy and infant mortality. Researchers at Dartmouth College and others have also found large differences in health spending per capita by region within the United States that are difficult to explain, and little or no indication that higher-spending regions achieve superior outcomes by spending more (Fisher et al. 2003a,b).

Understanding all the reasons for international and interregional differences is challenging and remains an active area of research. Nonetheless, in light of political realities and our budgetary situation, it seems safe to conclude that one way or another, the growth of per capita spending on health care will be bent downward relative to its long-run trend.

This chapter is not about predicting how we *will* reduce the growth of health care spending, nor is it an argument for a single magic solution that we should adopt to eliminate the problem. Reducing spending growth in a sensible way will surely involve a number of different strategies. I will focus on something I and many others think is one important component of the appropriate solution: changing the way that providers of health care are paid. More specifically, I will argue that we should move away from payment on a fee-for-service basis toward more "global" payment methods, paying provider organizations risk-adjusted but largely prospectively set amounts per enrollee.

Medicare is a leader in pursuing this sort of payment reform, through its experimentation with accountable care organizations (ACOs). Given Medicare's involvement as a government program, it is interesting to ask whether a movement toward global payment inevitably leads to a more highly regulated or even single-payer health care system, or whether it can be a step toward a more effective market-based system with a stronger role for competition and consumer choice. The issues get rather complex, but as I will discuss, I am somewhat optimistic that competition among ACOs (and other sorts of health insurance arrangements) is possible, and is indeed the most promising approach to making the market work better.

Bending the cost curve will continue to be very challenging. At the end of the chapter, I briefly discuss one issue I believe we will need to confront. Even if a well-designed competitive system is successful at eliminating truly wasteful spending, keeping the growth of spending at an acceptable level will require that we recognize and accept that not all care that offers any benefit, regardless of cost, should be provided.

BACKGROUND: HEALTH CARE MARKETS AND FEE-FOR-SERVICE

As a general rule, markets work well when consumers are freely spending their own money and can reasonably judge the quality of what they are buying. In that setting, producers compete to produce the things that consumers want, and to survive they must sell them at the lowest sustainable prices. A perennial question in health care economics is whether health care is different from other forms of economic activity in ways that have important implications for how well markets can work.

Early on, Kenneth Arrow (1963) clarified some of the most important peculiarities of health care markets, arising from the unpredictability of medical needs and the imbalance of technical knowledge between providers and consumers of care. Perhaps the most fundamental impediment to a textbook competitive market is that consumers want to be insulated from financial considerations when they are making decisions about health care for themselves or their loved ones, especially when the stakes are high and the circumstances are already stressful. In part this is ordinary risk aversion—a willingness to pay something (an insurance premium) to be protected from uncertain but potentially large bills that could arise from circumstances beyond one's control. But it is also a reflection of the conditions under which health care decisions are often made. It is perfectly rational, for example, to not want to think about money when making decisions about a spouse with cancer. As a result, while there can be an important role for consumer choice and consumer incentives in health care, consumers cannot be expected to constrain wasteful spending at the point of service in the same way they do in other markets.

While the rise of managed care in the 1990s promoted experimentation with different methods of payment to health care providers, fee-for-service remains the predominant way that they are paid. Alternatives to fee-for-service are most likely to be used by health maintenance organizations (HMOs), which cover a relatively small share of the population. For example, in 2015 only about 20 percent of Medicare enrollees were covered by HMOs (Jacobson et al. 2015). Among workers with employer-sponsored insurance, only 24 percent were in either HMOs or related but less restrictive point-of-service plans (Claxton et al. 2015). And even HMOs often use fee-for-service methods to pay providers.

Fee-for-service is the way we pay most other service providers that we deal with, be they lawyers, plumbers, or hairdressers, so why is it a problem in health care? A key difference with health care is that we are typically not the ones paying at the point of service, or we are paying only a small fraction of the total bill. Our doctors have a financial incentive to recommend more services as long as payment exceeds the marginal cost of production, and if we are insured we have little or no financial incentive to question their advice.

Other issues might have more to do with the way fee-for-service medicine is currently practiced and administered than with the method itself. Spending time with patients to evaluate their needs, counsel them about making lifestyle changes, or coordinate care among other doctors is generally not as well rewarded as running tests and performing procedures. Some valuable services are often not remunerated at all, such as a doctor communicating with a patient by phone or e-mail, or a nurse talking to a pharmacist about a patient's medications.

Perhaps we don't need to abandon fee-for-service, we just need to fix it, to pay for the right things at the right rates. But what would an ideal fee-for-service system look like? Congress and Medicare administrators devoted a lot of effort to answering that question back in the 1980s, when they worked to create a more rational system of payments to physicians. They commissioned a major study at Harvard University

(Hsiao et al. 1988) that arrived at the Resource Based Relative Value Scale (RBRVS), which was implemented in the early 1990s and, with modifications, is still in use today (Ginsburg 2012). The intent of the RBRVS is that payments for services be proportionate to the costs of producing them. The goal seems to be to create an environment that is "neutral" with regard to incentives, to let physicians' decisions be guided by clinical considerations rather than economic ones.

But the "cost" of a service is by no means unambiguously defined or easily measured. For example, for services that require equipment with high fixed costs, such as magnetic resonance imaging exams, the average cost per unit of service depends heavily on the volume of services, and average cost may diverge considerably from the economically relevant marginal cost. What cost should we be trying to match in setting a payment rate? The minimum average cost achieved by a provider operating at optimum capacity is one possible target (assuming we can determine what it is), but paying only that much might also undesirably limit patient access in geographic areas that cannot support the volume of services necessary to bring costs down to that level.[2] Paying more creates a profit opportunity that can lead to excessive use. To take another quite simple example, what is the cost of sending an e-mail to a patient? An e-mail requires some time and effort, which represents a real cost, but the amount of effort is hardly uniform across messages. Any flat rate per e-mail would leave payment unrelated to the effort expended.

Those involved with RBRVS know that it is difficult technically—and politically—to set payments in a neutral way (Ginsburg 2012). For example, the apparent bias in the payment system toward procedures and away from evaluation and management services—an issue that the RBRVS was intended to address from the beginning—remains a concern. I submit that in any fee-for-service system there will inevitably be services that are profitable at the margin and therefore encouraged, and other valuable services that cost more than they return in payment.

Furthermore, even if we could be neutral, a fee-for-service system has other shortcomings. If doctors can expect to be paid the reasonable cost of whatever services they provide, they have no positive financial incentive to maintain and improve the patient's health in the least costly way. When they are being paid for each service and the patient is not paying directly, they have no incentive to avoid costly but very low (or even zero) benefit care. One of the things that many doctors may like about fee-for-service is that it allows them to act as independent practitioners and doesn't *require* them to collaborate too closely with anyone else, but that is really a weakness from a social perspective. It is difficult to create incentives for collaboration under fee-for-service.

In a *New York Times* article, Bogdanich and McGinty (2011) provide an instructive example. When a patient undergoes a chest CT scan, it is very common for some hospitals to perform two scans consecutively, one without dye and the other with dye injected for contrast into the patient's veins. Radiologists say there is very rarely a clinical reason for doing consecutive scans, but in some hospitals when a chest scan is done, a second one follows more than 80 percent of the time. The aggregate amounts of money involved make this example almost trivial in the big picture of health care spending, and the extra payment may not have been the primary motivation for doing the second scan, but fee-for-service payment certainly does not discourage the practice. Of greater concern in this instance is that performing a second CT scan exposes the patient to additional radiation.

Fee-for-service payment systems can be made more rational, and government and private payers seek to do that all the time. Extra payments or penalties can be added for meeting or not meeting certain performance goals. Guidelines can be written that define the conditions under which particular services are reimbursable. Major capital investments can be subject to regulatory approval. But this also illustrates part of the problem with fee-for-service. Because of the perverse financial incentives that it creates, it requires these sorts of additional regulations—or one might say, micromanagement by payers—if spending growth is to be limited.

PAY FOR OUTPUT, NOT INPUT: BUNDLING

To an economist, the things that are reimbursed under a fee-for-service system—the well-baby visit, the flu shot, the MRI, or even the surgical repair of a damaged knee—are more like inputs than outputs. Individuals care about maintaining and improving health, and health care *services* are a means to that end. If it is possible to identify and pay more directly for outputs, then it seems preferable to do that. Paying for output appropriately should then make it possible to leave the decisions about inputs to the knowledgeable professionals and limit the amount of bureaucratic interference.

The principle of paying for output rather than input makes sense, but there are plenty of practical complications. A fundamental question is, what output should we pay for? One important idea that I will touch on only briefly is bundling by episode of care (Komisar, Feder, and Ginsburg 2011), which goes beyond payments for individual services to make a single payment for a package of care. Limited forms of bundling are already common in our system. For example, the diagnosis-related group payment system for inpatient hospital care that Medicare began using in the 1980s makes a single payment to a hospital for an admission based on the patient's diagnosis. Making a single payment to an obstetrician to cover prenatal care, delivery, and postpartum care is another kind of bundle. These examples stop short of bringing all providers of care (such as physicians and hospitals) into the same bundle, so they do not create incentives for collaboration across providers or for combining all the elements of care in an efficient way, as a more inclusive bundle might do.

One key issue with bundling is how to define an episode. Medicare is in the early stages of an initiative mandated by the Affordable Care Act called Bundled Payments for Care Improvement (BPCI). For the most part, BPCI defines episodes around certain types of inpatient admissions. It is working with several different bundling models, but some go well beyond the diagnosis-related group hospital payment system, in a positive direction, by defining the episode to begin prior to hospitalization and to extend for a period of time afterward, and by including all types of care in the same bundled payment (Cassidy 2015).

Some of the basic questions about bundling, such as how to deal with differences in severity across patients and how to reward quality of care, arise also with more global payment, which I will discuss next. For now I will suggest three reasons why bundling by episode seems less than ideal as the predominant way of paying for care. First, not all care can be readily grouped into episodes. Analyzing Medicare data, Cutler and Ghosh (2012) find that even if every inpatient stay and the outpatient services related to it are classified as part of an episode, only a little over half of program spending can be accounted for. A second and related point is that episode-based payment does not by itself create incentives to keep patients healthy so that episodes are avoided. Indeed, it may create financial incentives to organize care—or at least the way that care is reported—so as to *increase* the number of episodes. Third, if we wish to have a system in which incentives to optimize quality and cost are generated through the exercise of consumer choice, as in more standard market settings, episode-based payment may not be the best way to do so.[3]

COMPREHENSIVE CARE AS THE BASIS FOR PAYMENT

Good health is the output that we ultimately care about the most. We want the best care when episodes of ill health happen, but preventing them would be even better. Therefore, we might contemplate going beyond payment for episodes of care and consider making a single payment to an organization responsible for all of an individual's care.

This idea of paying health care organizations on a "capitation" basis, a fixed amount per person covered, is not new. Early examples of "prepaid group practice" in the United States go all the way back to the 1930s, and the most successful one developed into Kaiser Permanente, a health plan that today has more than 10 million enrollees nationwide. During the 1990s, payers and providers experimented rather extensively with capitation as a basis for payment, but a backlash against managed care led to a decline in its use in favor of a return to fee-for-service.

The backlash came from both consumers and doctors. For consumers, the big concern is that if providers incur costs but gain no additional revenue by providing more services, then they have an incentive to skimp on quality and to withhold costly but valuable care. For doctors, the main concerns depend on whether it is they, either individually or in groups, who are accepting capitation payments. If they are, then they may be taking on a great deal of risk for things that are beyond their control. What happens if a doctor enrolls a set of patients and an unusual fraction of them suffer costly illnesses or injuries despite the doctor's best efforts? Then the aggregate payment, which was expected to be adequate under normal circumstances, will not be sufficient to cover the cost of care.

With a large enough group of enrollees who are representative of the population from which they are drawn, the more or less random events that lead some people to incur high medical expenditures and others low can be expected to average out. Indeed, the ability to pool risks in a large population is what makes it possible for an insurance company to offer coverage at a price that people are willing to pay, without the insurance company itself being subject to excessive risk. But the population of patients that a single doctor, or even a group of doctors, is capable of serving may not be large enough to reduce the risk to an acceptable level.

Doctors and groups of doctors are understandably reluctant to accept capitation payment, especially full capitation, which makes them responsible for all the costs of a patient's care. If they work with an HMO or other organization that is itself accepting capitation payment and pays the doctors using fee-for-service, their concern becomes one of excessive pressure or interference from the HMO to limit costs.

The Accountable Care Organization Idea

Capitation remains a dirty word among many health care providers, and for many consumers the title HMO has negative connotations. A somewhat different idea and a new term has emerged among those who want to see providers accept responsibility for comprehensive care for defined populations. The title "Accountable Care Organization" (ACO) even made its way into the language of the Affordable Care Act.[4]

Section 3022 of the ACA discusses a Medicare Shared Savings Program that "promotes accountability for a patient population and coordinates items and services under parts A and B, and encourages investment in infrastructure and redesigned care processes for high quality and efficient service delivery." The act goes on to say that "groups of providers of services and suppliers . . . may work together to manage and coordinate care for Medicare fee-for-service beneficiaries through an accountable care organization." In 2015, 424 groups were participating as Medicare ACOs serving over 7.8 million beneficiaries (Cavanaugh 2014).

Advocates of ACOs take great pains to differentiate the concept from other forms of capitation payment. Four factors make ACOs different, based on the way Medicare is implementing the idea: 1) an ACO is usually an organization created and run by health care providers—no insurer middleman must come between Medicare and the clinicians or between the clinicians and enrollees; 2) payment involves the central idea of shared savings, which means that it is not in fact entirely fixed prospectively; 3) the amount of payment also depends on hitting certain quality targets; and 4) the Medicare enrollees linked to an ACO retain free choice of provider—they are not limited to receiving services from providers who are part of that ACO.

Many aspects of how Medicare's model of ACOs works are discussed elsewhere in more detail (for example, Berenson and Burton [2011]). I will focus on only a few points here, and in a somewhat simplified way. As noted above, an ACO participating with Medicare agrees to be accountable for the care of a population of Medicare enrollees. In the current model, enrollees do not actively choose an ACO but rather may be linked to one based on where they get their primary care. If the doctor providing the largest dollar amount of a particular enrollee's primary care (based on fee-for-service billings) is part of an ACO, then that enrollee is linked to that ACO.

The idea of shared savings warrants further explanation. Medicare sets a target amount of payment for the population covered by the ACO, but it actually continues to pay the ACO on a fee-for-service basis. The "savings" is the difference between the target and the total fee-for-service payments. Mathematically, a simple form of this system would look like this:

$$(4.1) \quad R = TOT_{FFS} + \alpha \times (TAR - TOT_{FFS}),$$

where R is total revenue for the ACO, TOT_{FFS} represents total fee-for-service payments, TAR is the target, and α is the "sharing rate." Note that in this formula the savings could be negative—if the fee-for-service billings exceeded the target—in which case the ACO would need to pay back a share (α) of the payments in excess of the target.[5]

Equation (4.1) may be rewritten as

$$(4.2) \quad R = \alpha \times TAR + (1 - \alpha) \times TOT_{FFS},$$

which shows that this payment mechanism is actually a combination of capitation and fee-for-service for values of α between 0 and 1. At one extreme ($\alpha = 1$) it is pure capitation, at the other ($\alpha = 0$) it is pure fee-for-service.

The hope, of course, is that the possibility of receiving shared savings will motivate the decision makers in the ACO to be more responsible for the costs of care, and to do things to reorganize care to reduce costs while maintaining or improving quality. So how is the decision about prescribing a particular service different in an ACO than as a fee-for-service practitioner? Under fee-for-service, the marginal financial gain or loss for providing a service is the difference between the fee and the marginal cost (MC) of providing the service, or simply

(4.3) $\text{Fee} - \text{MC}.$

As long as this expression is positive there is a financial incentive to provide the service. Things become more complicated in an ACO. There is still the fee, and the marginal cost is still incurred, but a share of the fee is taken back, and then there may be indirect effects. If providing better preventive care keeps a patient out of the hospital, for example, it reduces other costs that the organization would have incurred, but it also reduces fees that would have been earned on those other services. We can amend Expression (4.3) to read

(4.4) $\text{Fee} - \text{MC} - \alpha \times \text{Fee} + \text{indirect effects},$

recognizing that the indirect effects can themselves be complicated. If α is large (close to 1), then the fee for the service and for any services indirectly affected becomes less important, and financial incentives are more about direct costs of a service relative to costs that might be avoided by providing it, as would be the case in a true capitated system. An ACO should want to provide a service for which it is not directly reimbursed, as long as larger costs are thereby avoided.

While Expression (4.4) applies to the ACO as a whole, aligning the incentives of those actually making decisions about resource use, often individual doctors, is another matter. If clinicians continue to be paid mainly by fee-for-service, even if part of the fees are initially withheld, it will be no easy matter to get them to care about indirect savings they may create for the organization. It probably cannot be done well just by designing formulas for allocating shared savings among providers who are only minimally integrated. Successful ACOs will truly integrate providers across medical specialties with a shared purpose to coordinate care more effectively, and they will invest in shared information technology and in systems of data analysis to help them better understand their own performance.

ACOs: Regulation or Competition?

Having explained the basic ACO idea, I now discuss where it might take us if it catches on in a big way. Is the ACO model compatible with a greater reliance on market forces, with provider performance disciplined by the exercise of consumer choice, or is it better viewed as a form of incentive-based regulation? Given the growing interest in ACOs, along with ongoing discussion of the proper role of markets in health care, this is an important question in the debate over health care reform.

Because of the way ACOs are being implemented in Medicare, enrollees do not actively choose them. Enrollees can get linked to ACOs based on where they get their primary care, and in that way they can exercise a choice. It is certainly possible that an enrollee would choose a doctor because she belongs to an ACO with a reputation for high quality. But that choice has no implications for the enrollee's premium or for the services covered, nor is the enrollee limited to receiving services only from providers who are part of that ACO. Thus, the ACO's motivation for concern about *costs* (as opposed to quality) comes entirely from the incentives created by the payment mechanisms implemented by the regulator (Medicare). The possibility of using cost reductions to lower premiums and thereby attract more enrollees does not come into play.

ACO models are also attracting interest in private insurance markets (Higgins et al. 2011). One might suppose that if the model is being used in the private sector it must be part of a market approach. But consider the most prominent private example, the Alternative Quality Contract (AQC), created by Blue Cross Blue Shield (BCBS) of Massachusetts (Song et al. 2012). Groups of providers that participate in the AQC are similar in many ways to Medicare ACOs: they agree to accept responsibility for the comprehensive care of a group of enrollees, they can share in savings if they can keep total fee-for-service billings below a predetermined target, and they are rewarded for meeting quality goals.

The populations they are responsible for come from enrollees in the Massachusetts BCBS HMO. Each HMO enrollee must choose a primary care provider. If the provider is part of a group that is participating in the AQC, the enrollee is linked to that group. As in Medicare, an enrollee might well choose a doctor because he is part of a group with a reputation for high-quality care. But again, this choice has no implications for the premium the enrollee pays or the services covered. Thus, as in Medicare ACOs, incentives to control costs for groups participating in the AQC come from the payment model set up by BCBS. A group that does a superior job of controlling costs and could therefore afford to set lower premiums is precluded from using lower premiums to attract more enrollees.

So it seems that the ACO model, at least as it is currently being implemented by Medicare and in the AQC, is more a tool for changing provider incentives within a regulated system than a vehicle for empowering consumer choice. Can it be adapted in a way that would increase the role of consumers? I submit that it can, and that doing so would involve combining ACOs with an earlier idea called managed competition, most closely associated with economist Alain Enthoven (1993).

A Digression on Managed Competition

The aim of managed competition is to focus consumer choice around health plans rather than asking them to shop for individual services. Choice should then be organized in such a way that health plans set their own premiums, while individuals choosing among plans face the full difference in premiums between a higher- and lower-priced plan. Enthoven (1993) argued that in a properly designed competitive system, the health plans that would win out would be largely self-contained groups of providers: "Managed competition occurs at the level of integrated financing and delivery plans, not at the individual provider level. Its goal is to divide providers in each community into competing economic units and to use market forces to motivate them to develop efficient delivery systems" (p. 29). These "integrated delivery systems" would, in other words, look a lot like what we now call ACOs.[6]

There are several other important aspects of how competition is "managed" in this model. A health plan is required to accept all applicants during open enrollment periods. It must charge the same premium to all applicants for the same coverage (or only limited variation, perhaps by enrollee age, is allowed). The set of covered services and copayments are limited to a small number of different packages, to make consumer comparisons easier.

But because of prior differences in health status, some enrollees will cost much more to cover than others, regardless of what the health plan does. A key adjunct to these rules, therefore, is that payments to health plans be "risk adjusted," which means that plans that attract a sicker mix of enrollees are paid more, and plans that enroll a healthier mix are paid less. Without such risk adjustments, plans have strong incentives to do whatever they can to attract relatively healthy enrollees and avoid sicker ones, a frequent criticism of the way competition among health plans has traditionally operated. Risk adjustment is intended to help focus plan efforts on delivering the best product rather than on attracting the most profitable population. Risk adjustment is also a matter of fairness to plans and of making the managed competition approach acceptable to them. If plans are attempting to deliver high quality at a reasonable cost, they should not be penalized if they happen to attract a relatively unhealthy population.

The ideas of managed competition have been influential in U.S. health policy, and the ACA takes additional steps toward implementing them. Medicare already incorporates many of managed competition's features in two of its programs: Medicare Advantage (Medicare Part C) and the prescription drug benefit (Part D). Medicare Advantage (MA) is Medicare's program of capitation contracting with managed care plans, which has been around in different forms and under different names since the 1980s; the prescription drug benefit has only been available since 2006. Both programs have two key features: 1) Medicare makes risk-adjusted payments to participating health plans, and 2) plans make competitive bids that affect the premiums enrollees face; thus, plans can use their bids as a mechanism to attract enrollees.

The premium-setting processes and risk adjustment mechanisms are complicated in both programs (Duggan, Healy, and Morton 2008; Song, Cutler, and Chernew 2012). I will merely sketch the process used in MA. Each plan bids a premium it will accept for a person of average risk. These bids are compared with a county-specific benchmark rate determined by Medicare. If a bid is above the benchmark, then the difference is added to the enrollee's premium. As a result, the total premium received by the plan is equal to its bid. If the bid is below the benchmark, then the plan receives its bid plus 75 percent of the difference. However, the extra payment above the bid is to go back to enrollees in reduced premiums or added benefits. Medicare also adjusts the premium it pays to each plan based on the risk profile of the plan's enrollees, increasing the premium for a plan that attracts above-average risks and decreasing it for one with below-average risks. These risk adjustments are based on the enrollees' demographic characteristics and on diagnoses reported on their Medicare claims in the past year.

I would not suggest that the experience with either of these programs offers an unqualified endorsement for the merits of the managed competition model. If MA were really working well, it would be saving Medicare money relative to the traditional system, but that has not been the case. On the contrary, the Medicare Payment Advisory Commission has found that in recent years Medicare paid MA plans amounts that were significantly higher than it would have paid for the same enrollees in traditional Medicare. That made MA plans a target for rate reductions to help finance the coverage expansions contained in the ACA. As for Medicare Part D, it has in some ways performed better than critics expected (Duggan, Healy, and Morton 2008), but researchers analyzing actual plan choices have raised serious questions about the ability of many enrollees to choose plans in their own best interest (Abaluck and Gruber 2011; Heiss et al. 2013). These two programs demonstrate, nonetheless, that it is possible to use competitive bidding processes in Medicare—in other words, to allow participating health plans to set their own premiums—and it is fair to say that risk-adjustment mechanisms are getting more sophisticated over time.[7]

The ACA took a step toward broader application of the managed competition model by mandating the creation of "health insurance exchanges," institutions whereby individuals without employer-sponsored coverage or small businesses can shop for coverage, beginning in 2014.[8] These insurance exchanges have important managed competition features. For example, subsidies to individuals do not depend on the plan chosen, so that individuals bear the additional costs of choosing a more expensive plan. The exchanges also use risk adjustment to blunt incentives of plans to seek out the healthy and avoid the sick. A further example of a proposal to expand the application of managed competition is U.S. Representative and current House Speaker Paul Ryan's plan to convert Medicare to a program of "premium support," giving enrollees a fixed dollar amount that they could supplement as they wish and letting them shop for coverage. Ryan's original 2011 proposal would in effect have ultimately moved all enrollees into MA, but more recent versions of the plan retain traditional Medicare as an option that enrollees could choose (Feldman, Coulam, and Dowd 2012).[9]

Fitting ACOs into Managed Competition

Returning now to payment reform and in particular to ACOs, I would argue that the Medicare ACO model is not so different from the managed competition approach used in MA. If these two models are to converge, one important step is that enrollees must actively choose ACOs rather than merely be linked to them. One can understand the political motivation for making the introduction of ACOs as innocuous as possible for the Medicare population, but if we want consumer choice to help drive provider performance on both cost and quality, being served by an ACO must be a choice and it must have some consequences.[10] The enrollee should bear some cost in more limited access to providers, but the possibility of benefit through reduced premiums should also open up.[11]

The spending target for an ACO is initially being set by trending forward actual Medicare spending on the ACO's enrollees in the prior three-year period. Setting targets in this way is a form of risk adjustment—an ACO with enrollees who have used a lot of care in the past will have a higher target than one with enrollees who have used less care—and not so dissimilar to what is done in MA.[12] One could imagine altering the process of target setting to make it even more similar. An ACO could bid its own target for covering an enrollee of average risk, which would determine the premium that enrollees would pay, and then that bid amount could be risk-adjusted to determine the spending target that applied to that ACO.

The shared savings aspect of the ACO model does make it a little different from prospective payment as it operates in MA. We can highlight the difference by recalling our earlier equation for the revenue that an ACO receives:

$$(4.1) \quad R = TOT_{FFS} + \alpha \times (TAR - TOT_{FFS}).$$

A key issue is the value of α. With purely prospective payment, $\alpha = 1$, and once the target is set it is irrelevant what fee-for-service payments would have been. In the ACO model α can be a smaller number, such as 0.5, in which case revenues depend also on what they would have been under fee-for-service. Allowing revenues to depend also on TOT_{FFS} provides another form of risk adjustment, this one retrospective, in addition to that built into the determination of the target. Because enrollees' needs for services can be predicted only imperfectly based on information available prospectively, it will turn out that some ACOs will have enrollee populations that are sicker and more costly than expected, for reasons beyond the ACOs' control.

The drawback to setting $\alpha < 1$ is that it weakens the incentive to control costs and perpetuates to some degree the perverse incentives present in fee-for-service payment, because providing more services still adds to revenue. But there are important benefits to having shared savings and risks. They reduce the immediate financial benefit from withholding care that is present with purely prospective payment, which should be reassuring to enrollees. As noted, shared savings also reduce the risk faced by ACOs, which increases their willingness to participate, especially for smaller entities with more limited ability to themselves spread risk over large enrollee populations. Thus, the use of shared savings rather than purely prospective rates can be compatible with a market-based approach.[13]

The dependence of payments to ACOs on quality targets is also a departure from traditional capitation methodology, but Medicare is also introducing quality-based bonuses for MA plans, so this is not a fundamental difference. What about extending the ACO model outside Medicare to the nongovernment insurance market? Can it be done in a way that also relies on consumer choice to motivate provider groups to compete on both cost and quality? I am hopeful that it can, with health insurance exchanges used to manage the process.

I earlier noted a difficulty with the AQC model in Massachusetts. Enrollees attributed to a participating provider group are drawn from those in the BCBS HMO. But as in the Medicare ACO model, the enrollees do not actively choose a group, and their premiums and the set of covered services and available providers do not depend on the group to which they are linked. While enrollees may be drawn to a group on the basis of its reputation for quality, they get no direct benefit from choosing one that successfully controls costs. This situation could be remedied by having each provider group participating in the AQC act like a mini-HMO. Each group could have its own premium and its own set of in-network providers, and enrollees could choose among them. A shared savings approach, rather than relying only on prospectively set premiums, would reduce the risk borne by provider groups and make them more willing to participate in this sort of arrangement, as well as easing the fears of consumers about incentives to hold back care.

The obvious next question, though, is why would we need BCBS to mediate between consumers and provider groups? Why shouldn't consumers just choose the ACO directly? An entity is still needed to manage and administer the process, but for the most part a health insurance exchange is better suited to this task than a health insurer like BCBS. One important reason is that risk adjustment, which shifts premium revenues from insurance plans (or ACOs) that enroll relatively healthy populations to those that enroll more of the sick, should ideally be carried out over a pool that is as broad and representative as possible. The ACA did not extend health insurance exchanges beyond individual and small-firm coverage to the much larger pool of those insured through employment in large firms, but in the future we could move in that direction.

SUMMARY AND CONCLUSION

I began the chapter with a generally accepted claim that, at least in principle, the United States needs to bend the curve of health care spending rather substantially and rather soon. The greatest urgency comes from the burden of health care on government budgets, but any solution is likely to involve our entire health care system. Consumers and providers both must therefore be open to significant changes in the way our system works. Changing provider incentives by moving away from fee-for-service payment is one important step. Fee-for-service not only encourages the provision of any services that are profitable for providers without regard to their effectiveness, it contributes to the fragmented nature of our system and does not promote a focus on maintaining and improving health in the most cost-effective way.

The ACO idea—paying organizations of providers at largely prospective rates to be accountable for the care of defined populations—has a great deal of appeal. I have argued further that this approach can be consistent with using competitive bidding to set payment rates and relying on consumer choice to motivate ACOs to compete on both quality and cost. In essence, this is adapting the ACO model to the familiar idea of managed competition. We would need to move away from having individuals passively linked to ACOs and instead make membership an active choice, with consequences for premiums and provider networks. At the same time, in order to make managed competition more acceptable to somewhat smaller provider groups and to consumers, risk adjustments would be carried out not only prospectively but also retrospectively, as is already done in the Medicare prescription drug benefit. In other words, a shared savings model would be used rather than pure prospective payment. Making payments to ACOs (or other forms of health plans that consumers could alternatively choose) contingent on quality measures can also be a part of this model.

There are many important questions about whether the model I have outlined is a viable approach to significantly bending the curve of rising spending while promoting improvements in quality. In Medicare Advantage, for example, the managed competition model does not have a great track record of success (but the situation may be improving). Can incentives be made strong enough to motivate real change in the way medical practice is organized, real integration, without placing provider groups at too much risk (Frakt and Mayes 2012)? Is it reasonable to think that informed consumer choice can motivate good behavior by providers of something as complex as health coverage? Can we develop methods of risk adjustment that are fair to health plans and that eliminate the incentive to seek out certain types of enrollees while trying to avoid others? Will competition prove "workable" in the sense that combinations of providers will be unable to exercise excessive market power relative to consumers (Berenson et al. 2012; Quealy and Katz 2015)? The idea is promising enough that we should continue to move aggressively to get better answers to these questions.

In concluding the chapter, I want to briefly discuss one other issue that is relevant to how far we can potentially get in controlling health spending through a market-based strategy. I will first talk about it in a simplified, very abstract way, and then relate things in a more practical way to Medicare Part D. Let the curve in Figure 4.3 represent the relationship between health spending and health if resources were being used in the most effective way—a kind of "production function" relating inputs to output in an efficient manner. Points B and C, for example, are both on the production function; moving from B to C involves increasing spending—giving up more of other things—to get improved health.

Many analysts say that we do not have to think about trade-offs between health and other things because the poor incentives built into our system actually leave us at a point like A, beneath the production function. If so, improving incentives might reduce spending and improve health simultaneously, moving us, for example, from A to B. But if we can get to point B, the question of where we want to be along the curve must ultimately involve trade-offs.[14]

In other market situations, when purchasing cars, televisions, or cell phones, for example, people face trade-offs between cost and quality all the time. Generally, we are happy to let them make their own decisions. Ability to pay matters, people with higher incomes drive nicer cars, but we are typically fine with that as an intrinsic part of a free enterprise system. Applying the same logic to health care, we might think of the curve in Figure 4.3 at the level of one individual, and of the points along the curve as different insurance packages that have both different premiums and levels of coverage, including different sets of services that are covered. We hope that market forces will eliminate packages that lie below the curve. Then individuals can choose where along the curve they want to be, say, at point B or C. Naturally, the wealthier will find it easier to pay for C and will be more likely to choose it.

But are we as a society willing to live with that? Will a Medicare program that explicitly lets the rich buy access to services that the poor cannot afford be acceptable, or will it be seen as inappropriate rationing? As things stand, the Medicare program does not explicitly consider costs when it makes decisions about whether new services will be covered. Similarly, the ACA established the Patient-Centered Outcomes Research Institute to study the comparative effectiveness of different

Figure 4.3 Eliminating Waste versus Facing Trade-offs

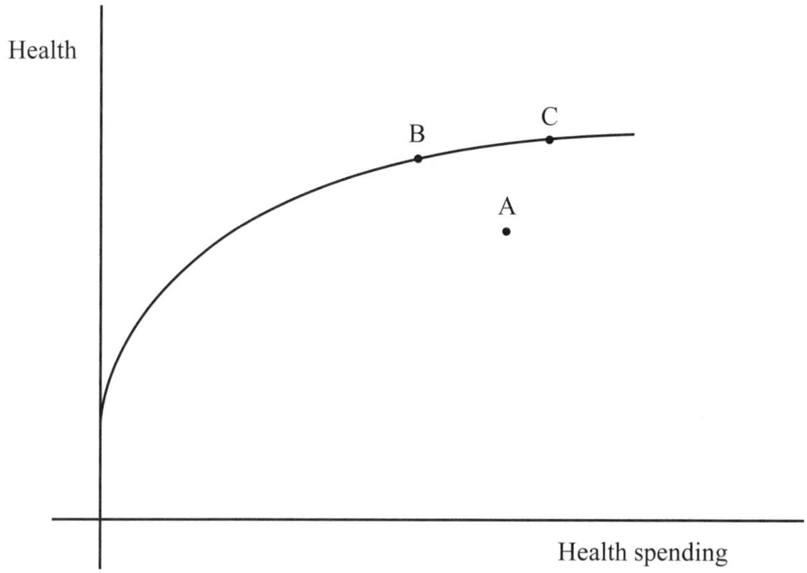

medical interventions, but it prohibited Medicare from using analyses of cost per quality-adjusted life year to make coverage decisions.

The example of Medicare Part D is instructive. Part D drug plans are not required to cover every drug. In many therapeutic classes, a plan can give preferred status (assign lower copayments) to certain drugs relative to others that are close therapeutic substitutes. This gives a plan leverage to negotiate with drug manufacturers for lower prices, the savings from which (one hopes) would as a result of competition largely be passed along to enrollees in lower premiums. However, the ability of plans to differentiate themselves through the set of drugs they cover is limited. They are required to cover at least two drugs in every therapeutic class, and "all or substantially all" drugs in six protected classes (immunosuppressants, antidepressants, antipsychotics, anticonvulsants, HIV antiretrovirals, and cancer). As Duggan, Healy, and Morton (2008) discuss, these restrictions limit the ability of plans to negotiate with manufacturers over prices. They also limit a plan's ability to keep premiums low by choosing not to cover certain high-cost drugs of limited or questionable benefit.

A similar issue arises with respect to insurance plans offered in health insurance exchanges. When individuals are mandated to have insurance coverage, some minimum standard of what constitutes creditable coverage must be set. The more inclusive that standard, the less scope there is for individuals to make trade-offs to get lower premiums. Similarly, the set of services that an ACO is accountable for providing must be defined. The main point is that eliminating truly wasteful spending from the system (getting from point A to the curve in Figure 4.3), as difficult as that is to achieve, will not be enough to limit spending growth to an acceptable level in the long run. As a society we must be willing to face the possibility that small benefits in health care may sometimes come at too high a cost.

Notes

1. By "excess cost growth," the CBO means the amount by which the growth of health spending per capita, adjusted for changes in the age composition of the population, exceeds the growth of the economy's capacity to produce on a per capita basis.
2. The Medicare Payment Advisory Commission (MedPAC) advises Congress about Medicare and generally does excellent work. Chapter 2 of its June 2011 report (MedPAC 2011) is entitled "Improving Payment Accuracy and Appropriate Use of Ancillary Services." It is interesting that the chapter refers to "payment accuracy" more than 25 times but never defines what "accuracy" means.
3. Porter and Teisberg (2007) would disagree. See Note 6.
4. Although many researchers have contributed to the development of this idea, the person most associated with it is Elliot Fisher, a physician and researcher at Dartmouth. Fisher says that the term emerged originally in discussion between him and Glenn Hackbarth, former chair of MedPAC. Health policy discussions abound with three-letter abbreviations. In this chapter, the most prominent and easily confused are ACO, for Accountable Care Organization, and ACA, for Affordable Care Act, the short title of the health care reform passed in 2010. Adding to the confusion, I will later discuss the AQC, or Alternative Quality Contract, a way of contracting with ACO-like entities developed by Blue Cross Blue Shield of Massachusetts.
5. Although I will frame the discussion around Equation (1), Medicare has in fact introduced several variations of the ACO model, including Pioneer (for organizations that are more prepared to take on risk based on prior experience with doing so) and two tracks in the Shared Savings Program (Berenson and Burton 2011). All of them involve a range in the neighborhood of the target where $\alpha = 0$, meaning that the organization is effectively paid fee-for-service. In track 1 of the

Shared Savings Program, α = 0 in the first three years whenever TOT_{FFS} exceeds the target—the organization initially bears no downside risk. In 2015 Medicare announced that organizations in track 1 would be allowed to stay there for an additional three years. It also established a track 3 for organizations willing to accept greater risk.

6. Porter and Teisberg (2007) offer a different vision of competition. They argue that medical providers are best organized into "integrated practice units" focused around particular "medical conditions and cycles of care." These entities would be well positioned to accept bundled payments for episodes or "cycles" of care. Arguably, rather than relying on single entities responsible for all types of care, organizing groups around particular conditions could lead to gains from greater specialization and more opportunity for choice. But how these ideas could be integrated into a model of insurance and cost-conscious consumer choice does not seem to be well worked out. One could imagine an insurance plan that in return for a premium covers primary care and also provides in effect a set of vouchers for treatment of particular conditions as they arise. If you have diabetes, are diagnosed with breast cancer, or experience severe low back pain, you have a voucher that covers standard quality care for that condition over a defined episode or for some defined period of time. If you want to use a group that charges more than the voucher covers, you pay the difference. I am not aware of any real-world examples of such a model of health insurance. For further discussion see Enthoven, Crosson, and Shortell (2007).
7. Brown et al. (2014), however, find that MA insurers may be a step ahead of the program administrators. They find that even after Medicare made changes in 2004 to better capture differences in risk across enrollees, MA plans were still attracting relatively healthy enrollees conditional on measured risk. On the other hand, working with a larger data set, Newhouse et al. (2014) do not replicate those findings, and on the whole they are more optimistic about the future of managed competition in MA.
8. Participation in the exchange for small businesses has been much slower to develop than exchange participation by individuals (Galewitz 2015).
9. The original Ryan plan for Medicare was strongly criticized by Democrats. For example, in his acceptance speech for the 2012 presidential nomination, President Obama, referring to the Ryan plan, said, "I will never turn Medicare into a voucher." However, much (though certainly not all) of the criticism of the plan had to do with the way that the premium support (or voucher) amount would be set and updated over time, with critics arguing the plan would shift very substantial costs to enrollees. In principle, the level of premium support is a separable issue from the concept itself.
10. One analyst stated, accurately, that "proponents of the shared savings model have designed an approach that attempts to upset or dislocate no one" (Berenson 2010).
11. Improving consumer incentives is not the only reason for asking that enrollees in an ACO be limited to the set of providers affiliated with it. An ACO faces additional risk that it will have little ability to control if it is accountable for Medicare services that an enrollee receives from providers outside the ACO.

12. Risk adjustment in MA is based on enrollee demographic characteristics and past diagnoses rather than directly on past spending, but the weights applied to the variables that go into the risk adjustment are based on how those variables predict spending in traditional Medicare. Setting a target based on the past spending experience of a group's own enrollees could have the perverse effect of penalizing groups that were already managing care efficiently by giving them lower targets.
13. After-the-fact risk adjustment (or shared savings and risks, which essentially is the same thing) is already present in Medicare Part D. If a prescription drug plan's expenses for drugs are more than 5 percent above or below its target based on risk-adjusted premiums, Medicare shares in the cost overrun or the savings (Duggan, Healy, and Morton 2008). A similar approach is being used during the first three years of operation of health insurance exchanges under the ACA, although funding has been less than insurers anticipated (Blase 2015; Cunningham 2012). Interestingly, however, in Part D and in the insurance exchanges the insurance plan accepts full risk in the vicinity of the target ($\alpha = 1$), whereas with ACOs the opposite is the case, $\alpha = 0$ in the vicinity of the target (see also Note 5).
14. Over time the entire curve shifts upward as a result of advances in knowledge (although other factors, such as worsening diets, may work to shift it down). But new knowledge also extends the relatively flat part of the curve by expanding our capacity to spend large amounts of money for small expected benefits.

References

Abaluck, Jason, and Jonathan Gruber. 2011. "Heterogeneity in Choice Inconsistencies among the Elderly: Evidence from Prescription Drug Plan Choice." *American Economic Review* 101(3): 377–381.

Arrow, Kenneth J. 1963. "Uncertainty and the Welfare Economics of Medical Care." *American Economic Review* 53(5): 941–997.

Berenson, Robert A. 2010 "Shared Savings Program for Accountable Care Organizations: A Bridge to Nowhere?" *American Journal of Managed Care* 16(10): 721–726.

Berenson, Robert A., and Rachel A. Burton. 2011. "Accountable Care Organizations in Medicare and the Private Sector: A Status Update." Washington, DC: Urban Institute.

Berenson, Robert A., Paul B. Ginsburg, Jon B. Christianson, and Tracy Yee. 2012. "The Growing Power of Some Providers to Win Steep Payment Increases from Insurers Suggests Policy Remedies May Be Needed." *Health Affairs* 31(5): 973–981.

Blase, Brian. 2015. "New Data Shows Large Insurer Losses on Obamacare Plans." *Forbes*, October 12. http://www.forbes.com/sites/theapothecary/2015/10/12/new-data-shows-large-insurer-losses-on-obamacare-plans/ (accessed December 20, 2015).

Bogdanich, Walt, and Jo Craven McGinty. 2011. "Medicare Claims Show Overuse for CT Scanning." *New York Times*, June 18, A:1.

Brown, Jason, Mark Duggan, Ilyana Kuziemko, and William Woolston. 2014. "How Does Risk Selection Respond to Risk Adjustment? Evidence from the Medicare Advantage Program." *American Economic Review* 104(10): 3335–3364.

Cassidy, Amanda. 2015. "Health Policy Brief: Bundled Payments for Care Improvement Initiative." *Health Affairs*, November 23. http://www.healthaffairs.org/healthpolicybriefs/brief.php?brief_id=148 (accessed December 18, 2015).

Cavanaugh, Sean. 2014. "ACOs Moving Ahead." *The CMS Blog*. http://blog.cms.gov/2014/12/22/acos-moving-ahead/ (accessed December 18, 2015).

Claxton, Gary, Matthew Rae, Michelle Long, Nirmita Panchal, Anthony Damico, Kevin Kenward, and Heidi Whitmore. 2015. "Employer Health Benefits: 2015 Annual Survey." Menlo Park, CA: Henry J. Kaiser Foundation and Chicago: Health Research & Educational Trust.

Congressional Budget Office. 2015. "The 2015 Long-Term Budget Outlook." Washington, DC: Congressional Budget Office. https://www.cbo.gov/publication/50250 (accessed September 4, 2015).

Cunningham, Rob. 2012. "Health Policy Brief: Risk Adjustment in Health Insurance." *Health Affairs*, August 30. http://www.healthaffairs.org/healthpolicybriefs/brief.php?brief_id=74 (accessed December 21, 2015).

Cutler, David M., and Kaushik Ghosh. 2012. "The Potential for Cost Savings through Bundled Episode Payments." *New England Journal of Medicine* 366(12): 1075–1077.

Duggan, Mark, Patrick Healy, and Fiona Scott Morton. 2008. "Providing Prescription Drug Coverage to the Elderly: America's Experiment with Medicare Part D." *Journal of Economic Perspectives* 22(4): 69–92.

Enthoven, Alain C. 1993. "The History and Principles of Managed Competition." *Health Affairs* 12 Suppl: 24–48.

Enthoven, Alain C., Francis J. Crosson, and Stephen M. Shortell. 2007. "'Redefining Health Care': Medical Homes or Archipelagos to Navigate?" *Health Affairs* 26(5): 1366–1372.

Feldman, Roger, Robert Coulam, and Bryan Dowd. 2012. "Competitive Bidding Can Help Solve Medicare's Fiscal Crisis." *AEI Health Policy Outlook*, no. 2, February. Washington, DC: American Enterprise Institute.

Fisher, Elliott S., David E. Wennberg, Therese A. Stukel, Daniel J. Gottlieb, F. L. Lucas, and Étoile L. Pinder. 2003a. "The Implications of Regional Variations in Medicare Spending. Part 1: The Content, Quality, and Accessibility of Care." *Annals of Internal Medicine* 138(4): 273–287.

———. 2003b. "The Implications of Regional Variations in Medicare Spending. Part 2: Health Outcomes and Satisfaction with Care." *Annals of Internal Medicine* 138(4): 288–298.

Frakt, Austin B., and Rick Mayes. 2012. "Beyond Capitation: How New Payment Experiments Seek to Find the 'Sweet Spot' in Amount of Risk Providers and Payers Bear." *Health Affairs* 31(9): 1951–1958.

Galewitz, Phil. 2015. "Small Businesses Snub Obamacare's SHOP Exchange." *Kaiser Health News*, November 5. http://khn.org/news/small-businesses-snub-obamacares-shop-exchange/ (accessed December 21, 2015).

Ginsburg, Paul B. 2012. "Fee-For-Service Will Remain a Feature of Major Payment Reforms, Requiring More Changes in Medicare Physician Payment." *Health Affairs* 31(9): 1977–1983.

Hall, Robert E., and Charles I. Jones. 2007. "The Value of Life and the Rise in Health Spending." *Quarterly Journal of Economics* 122(1): 39–72.

Heiss, Florian, Adam Leive, Daniel McFadden, and Joachim Winter. 2013. "Plan Selection in Medicare Part D: Evidence from Administrative Data." *Journal of Health Economics* 32(6): 1325–1344.

Higgins, Aparna, Kristin Stewart, Kristin Dawson, and Carmella Bocchino. 2011. "Early Lessons from Accountable Care Models in the Private Sector: Partnerships between Health Plans and Providers." *Health Affairs* 30(9): 1718–1727.

Hsiao, William C., Peter Braun, Daniel Dunn, Edmund R. Becker, Margaret DeNicola, and Thomas R. Ketcham. 1988. "Results and Policy Implications of the Resource-Based Relative-Value Study." *New England Journal of Medicine* 319(13): 881–888.

Jacobson, Gretchen, Anthony Damico, Tricia Neuman, and Marsha Gold. 2015. "Medicare Advantage 2015 Spotlight: Enrollment Market Update." Menlo Park, CA: The Henry J. Kaiser Foundation. https:// http://kff.org/medicare/issue-brief/medicare-advantage-2015-spotlight-enrollment-market-update/ (accessed December 18, 2015).

Keehan, Sean P., Gigi A. Cuckler, Andrea M. Sisko, Andrew J. Madison, Sheila D. Smith, Devin A. Stone, John A. Poisal, Christian J. Wolfe, and Joseph M. Lizonitz. 2015. "National Health Expenditure Projections, 2014–24: Spending Growth Faster than Recent Trends." *Health Affairs* 34(8): 1407–1417.

Komisar, Harriet L., Judy Feder, and Paul B. Ginsburg. 2011. *"Bundling" Payment for Episodes of Hospital Care*. Washington, DC: Center for American Progress.

Medicare Payment Advisory Commission (MedPAC). 2011. *Medicare and the Health Care Delivery System*. Report to Congress, June. Washington, DC: MedPAC.

Newhouse, Joseph P., Mary Price, J. Michael McWilliams, John Hsu, and Thomas G. McGuire. 2014. "How Much Favorable Selection Is Left in Medicare Advantage?" NBER Working Paper No. 20021. Cambridge, MA: National Bureau of Economic Research.

Porter, Michael E., and Elizabeth Olmsted Teisberg. 2007. "How Physicians Can Change the Future of Health Care." *Journal of the American Medical Association* 297(10): 1103–1111.

Quealy, Kevin, and Margot Sanger Katz. 2015. "The Experts Were Wrong about the Best Places for Better and Cheaper Health Care." *New York Times*, December 15. http://www.nytimes.com/interactive/2015/12/15/upshot/the-best-places-for-better-cheaper-health-care-arent-what-experts-thought.html?rref=upshot&_r=0 (accessed January 12, 2016).

Song, Zirui, David M. Cutler, and Michael E. Chernew. 2012. "Potential Consequences of Reforming Medicare into a Competitive Bidding System." *Journal of the American Medical Association* 308(5): 459–460.

Song, Zirui, Dana Gelb Safran, Bruce E. Landon, Mary Beth Landrum, Yulei He, Robert E. Mechanic, Matthew P. Day, and Michael E. Chernew. 2012. "The 'Alternative Quality Contract,' Based on a Global Budget, Lowered Medical Spending and Improved Quality." *Health Affairs* 31(8): 1885–1894.

5
The Potential Effects of the Affordable Care Act on Disability Insurance and Workers' Compensation

Marcus Dillender
W.E. Upjohn Institute for Employment Research

The passage of the Affordable Care Act (ACA) represents one of the largest overhauls to the United States health care system since the introduction of Medicare and Medicaid. Among the reform's many provisions are an employer mandate, an individual mandate, an expansion of Medicaid, subsidies for low-income people to purchase coverage, and the establishment of health insurance exchanges. The ACA also reforms the individual market and implements many measures aimed at reducing medical costs.

Despite its many changes to the health care system, the ACA largely ignores related social insurance programs that also provide health care. Two programs in particular—federal disability and workers' compensation—deal with people with medical issues and have overlapping agendas with health insurance. Disability insurance provides health insurance for people who are unable to work for over a year due to health concerns, while workers' compensation insurance pays medical expenses for people injured at work. Unlike traditional health insurance, both programs also provide cash assistance to beneficiaries.

Although the ACA does not address these programs, it could have potentially major spillover effects on both federal disability and workers' compensation. First, the ACA could affect the likelihood that people apply for these programs since health insurance may substitute for the types of services they provide. This would affect the number and types of people receiving benefits as well as overall costs. Second, the ACA has several features that will change the types of insurance plans people have, such as eliminating copays for preventive care and taxing expensive, high-benefit plans. These features could result in healthier people or more cost shifting. Finally, the ACA implements many changes that alter medical resources. Since both disability and workers' compensation tap into the same systems as health insurance, changes that affect the medical system more generally will affect these programs as well.

This chapter discusses the implications that the ACA has for federal disability insurance and workers' compensation insurance. I do not attempt to determine whether the net impact of the costs of these programs will be positive or negative, as there is much uncertainty about the implementation and impact of the ACA. Instead, I discuss various aspects of the ACA, federal disability insurance, and workers' compensation, and I consider the possible interactions between the ACA and these social insurance programs.

THE AFFORDABLE CARE ACT

Implementation of the ACA began immediately after it was signed into law in 2010 and will continue until 2020. Table 5.1 summarizes various aspects of the law.

The employer mandate requires that companies with 50 or more full-time employees offer affordable coverage to their full-time employees or pay a penalty. The penalty for not offering health insurance is $2,000 per employee after the first 30 employees. Employers' plans must pay for at least 60 percent of covered health care expenses, and employees must pay no more than 9.5 percent of family income for the coverage. To prevent employers from offering plans that meet these requirements but do not meet employees' needs, the ACA also assesses firms that offer coverage a separate penalty of $3,000 for each employee who receives subsidized coverage through the exchanges.

The individual mandate requires nearly everyone to have health insurance or pay a penalty. The penalty for not having health insurance eventually rises to the maximum of $695 per uninsured person or 2.5 percent of household income over the filing threshold. To avoid the penalty, nonexempt individuals must maintain minimum essential coverage, which is defined as employer-sponsored coverage, government-sponsored coverage, or coverage purchased through the individual marketplace. Everyone is subject to the mandate except the following groups: people with incomes below 100 percent of the federal poverty level, people not required to file income taxes, people with religious objections, American Indians, undocumented immigrants, and incarcerated persons.

In addition to requiring that individuals purchase insurance, the ACA also established health insurance exchanges. These marketplaces opened in 2013 and allow people to compare plans from the individual market on a single website. The ACA issued several reforms for the individual market as well, including requiring insurers to accept all who apply for coverage, restricting the number of factors that could be used for pricing, and requiring certain coverage. To make insurance more affordable for people whose employers do not offer insurance and who are ineligible for Medicaid, the ACA provides subsidies for those making up to 400 percent of the federal poverty level.

In addition to subsidizing coverage for people not eligible for Medicaid, the ACA originally required that states expand Medicaid so that all households with incomes below 133 percent of the federal poverty level would qualify. The federal government would pay for the full cost of these newly eligible people in the first three years and no less than 90 percent thereafter. However, in June 2012, the Supreme Court ruled that the federal government could not require states to expand their Medicaid coverage; thus, the expansion of Medicaid is optional (Kaiser Family Foundation 2012). As of July 2014, 26 states and the District of Columbia have opted to expand Medicaid (Kaiser Family Foundation 2014).

The ACA also implements a variety of measures aimed at reducing Medicare costs. It has established the Independent Payment Advisory Board (IPAB), which will make recommendations to cut Medicare costs if they grow larger than the per capita GDP plus one percentage point. If Congress fails to pass an alternative proposal with the same cost savings, the IPAB recommendations will become law. The IPAB can also make nonbinding recommendations about private health spending. In addition to the IPAB, the ACA also encourages physicians and hospitals to form accountable care organizations (ACOs), which are sets of providers that bear responsibility for the cost and quality of care delivered to Medicare patients. Any Medicare savings from this coordinated

Table 5.1 Summary of Major Changes under the Affordable Care Act

Employer mandate	
Provisions	Employers with 50 or more full-time employees must offer a health insurance plan to all full-time employees or pay an annual penalty.[a,b]
Full-time definition	30 or more hours per week[b]
Penalties	Two types of penalties:
	• Must pay $2,000 per full-time employee (after first 30 employees) for not offering any insurance options
	• Must pay $3,000 for not offering affordable coverage, for all employees receiving a tax credit for insurance purchased on exchange[a,b]
Contribution requirement	Insurance plan must pay for at least 60% of covered health care expenses for a typical population, and employees must pay no more than 9.5% of family income for employer coverage.[a]
Individual mandate	
Provisions	All people must purchase health insurance or pay a penalty.
Penalty for not buying	The penalty is the greater of
	• For 2014, $95 per uninsured person or 1% of household income over the filing threshold
	• For 2015, $325 per uninsured person or 2% of household income over the filing threshold
	• For 2016 and beyond, $695 per uninsured person or 2.5% of household income over the filing threshold.[b]
Subsidized insurance	For anyone earning up to 400% of poverty level whose employer does not offer health insurance, covers less than 60% of the actuarial value, or whose employee share exceeds 9.5% of income.[a]

Exemptions	Income below 100% of the federal poverty level; not being required to file income taxes; having religious objections; having a coverage gap shorter than three months; or being an American Indian, undocumented immigrant, or incarcerated person.[a]
Medicaid	
To qualify	Expanded so that people with a household income below 133% of the poverty level will qualify.[a]
Individual market	
Can charge different premiums based on	Family structure, geography, age, and tobacco use.[a]
Guaranteed issue	Yes[a]
Marketplaces created	State Exchanges, which allow individuals and small businesses to compare and purchase private insurance that meets coverage standards.[a]

SOURCE: [a]Kaiser Family Foundation (2013); [b]Kolstad and Kowalski (2012).

care would be shared with providers. Additionally, the ACA reduces Medicare payments to hospitals with high rates of potentially preventable readmissions. In doing so, it alters hospitals' incentives to provide high-quality and cost-effective care on the first admission. Finally, the ACA increases the government's resources to fight fraud, which could save money, since the Congressional Budget Office estimates that each additional dollar spent on fraud prevention reduces $1.75 of Medicare spending (Zuckerman 2010).

As they were intended to do, these reforms have increased health insurance coverage. By June 2014, around 10.3 million more adults had health insurance because of the ACA (Sommers et al. 2014). This number is expected to grow over the next several years. The Congressional Budget Office and the Joint Committee on Taxation predict that the ACA will result in 19 million people having insurance in 2015 who otherwise would not. They expect this number to increase to 26 million by 2017 (Congressional Budget Office 2014). The anticipated cost of the ACA net of any savings is $1,383 billion for 2015–2024. The vast majority of these costs come from increased spending on Medicaid, as well as subsidies for people purchasing insurance in the marketplace. Schoen et al. (2011) estimate that the ACA could lead to a 70 percent decrease in the underinsurance rate, while Hill (2012) estimates that the ACA will reduce out-of-pocket spending for people with individual insurance.

FEDERAL DISABILITY INSURANCE

Basic Program Information

Federal disability insurance pays benefits to people under the full retirement age who are unable to work because they have a medical condition that is expected to last at least one year or result in death. Disabled people are potentially eligible for two different programs: Social Security Disability Insurance (SSDI) and Supplemental Security Income (SSI). The SSDI program provides benefits to individuals who have paid into the Social Security system and meet certain minimum work requirements, and the SSI program is means tested and does not have work or contribution requirements, but it restricts benefits to individuals with certain asset and resource limitations (Moulta-Ali 2013).

With SSDI, the benefit amount is related to the disabled worker's former earnings in covered employment. The average benefit amount as of 2012 was $1,130 for disabled workers (Social Security Administration 2013). SSDI recipients can receive health insurance coverage through Medicare but only after a two-year waiting period that begins the day they qualify for benefits. After a disabling event, individuals must wait at least five months before receiving cash benefits.

The SSI program pays a flat cash benefit to aged, blind, and disabled individuals who have very limited income and assets. The benefit amount for SSI as of 2012 was $698 for eligible individuals and $1,048 for eligible couples (Social Security Administration 2014a). Individuals on SSI receive health insurance through the Medicaid program. Unlike SSDI recipients, SSI recipients receive cash benefits and health insurance immediately upon qualifying for benefits. As of 2012, around 86 percent of the people receiving SSI benefits were disabled (Center on Budget and Policy Priorities 2014).

Figure 5.1 shows the number of SSDI recipients, including dependents and the money spent on SSDI over time. The number of people on federal disability has swelled in recent decades. In 1970, approximately 2.7 million people, or about 1.3 percent of the population received SSDI. By the end of 2012, approximately 10.9 million people, or 3.5 percent of the population, received SSDI. Total SSDI benefits paid in 2012 were $137 billion (Social Security Administration 2013). Autor and Duggan (2006) find that this rapid increase in the number of people receiving SSDI can be attributed to congressional reforms to disability screening that enabled workers with low mortality disorders to more easily qualify for benefits, a rise in the after-tax SSDI benefit, and an increase in female labor force participation, which expanded the pool of eligible workers.

Figure 5.2 shows SSI applicants and new recipients over time. While the number of people newly receiving SSI because of their age has decreased slightly over time, the number of new disabled recipients has increased. As of 2012, around 8.3 million people received SSI, while total SSI benefits paid were $49 billion (Social Security Administration 2013).

Figure 5.1 SSDI Beneficiaries and Benefits by Year

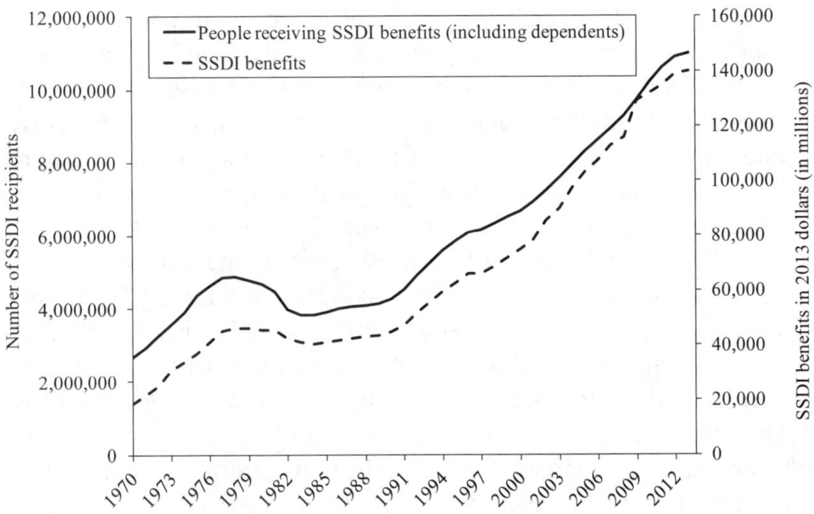

SOURCE: Social Security Administration (2014c).

Social Security and Medicare are both funded from a 15.3 percent payroll tax on earnings that is split equally between employees and employers. Of the 15.3 percent, 1.8 percent of the payroll tax goes into the disability trust fund to pay for SSDI, and 2.9 percent goes toward Medicare; the rest of the tax goes in the Old Age and Survivors Insurance Fund (Moulta-Ali 2013). SSI is financed through the general revenue of the United States. Medicaid, which SSI recipients receive, is funded jointly by state and federal government.

The ACA's Potential Effect on Disability Insurance

The ACA will likely exert two countervailing forces on people's decisions to apply for disability insurance. Applicants to both SSDI and SSI face uncertainty about whether or not they qualify for benefits, and they may have to wait long periods of time for their disability status to be determined. During this time, applicants cannot work. Since employer-sponsored insurance has traditionally been better than the other forms of insurance available, people may have had to go without

Figure 5.2 SSI Applicants and New Recipients by Year

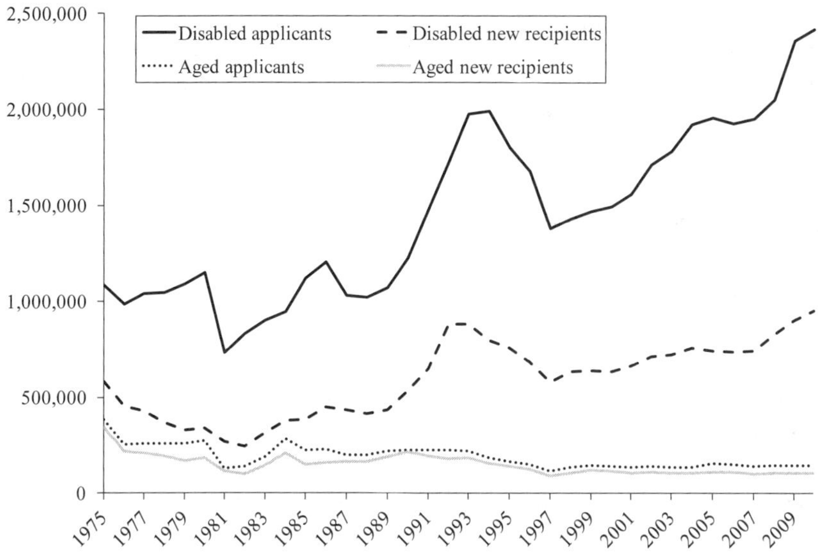

SOURCE: Social Security Administration (2014d).

high-quality, affordable health insurance to apply for disability coverage. However, the insurance exchanges and subsidized coverage from the ACA promise affordable health insurance outside employment. Similarly, the ACA mandates that insurance companies accept all who apply, which will increase coverage options for those with a disability. Improving coverage options for those with a disability could free workers from employment lock, thereby reducing the costs of applying for disability coverage. This would cause the number of disability applications to rise, especially those for SSDI, since those applicants will have to wait an additional two years after receiving benefits before they receive Medicare coverage. On the other hand, a lack of good health insurance alternatives to employer-sponsored health insurance is one reason people apply for SSDI. By creating good health insurance opportunities apart from employer-sponsored coverage and Medicare, the ACA lowers the benefit of applying for disability. This could result in fewer people applying for disability.

Two papers empirically examine which effect dominates. Gruber and Kubik (2002) study how health insurance factors into the likelihood that people apply for SSDI using Health and Retirement Study data. They find that people who have access to insurance from a source other than their own employers, such as insurance through a spouse's employer or retiree coverage, are 26–74 percent more likely to apply for SSDI benefits than those without such alternative sources of coverage.

Maestas, Mullen, and Strand (2014) study what happened to disability applications after the Massachusetts health insurance reform, which has a structure that is very similar to the ACA. They find that disability applications increased in Massachusetts relative to neighboring states in the first year following health insurance reform. After the first year, there was no statistically significant effect of the reform on total applications. These results suggest that there may have been pent-up demand for disability benefits for people who had been working with impairments. Despite finding no evidence of long-term changes in the aggregate, they find important county-level heterogeneity. They find that SSDI and SSI applications increased in counties with high levels of health insurance coverage prior to the reform and decreased in counties with low levels of coverage. Since Massachusetts had higher insurance coverage than the rest of the country before its health insurance reform, Maestas, Mullen, and Strand conclude that the ACA may lead to a net decrease in disability insurance applications.

Just as the need for health insurance has resulted in some people being tied to employers, it can lead to some people being tied to disability insurance. Coe and Rupp (2013) examine how access to health insurance for disabled individuals in both the nongroup market and Medicaid affects the exit from disability. They find that SSI beneficiaries with some Medicaid expenditures are more likely to exit disability when they have more health insurance options available to them, as are SSDI recipients who do not have access to supplemental health insurance outside Medicare.

Gruber and Kubik (2002) suggest that the ACA would lead to an increase in disability applicants. However, results from the Massachusetts reform suggest that the ACA will likely affect certain people and areas differently than others. The results of Coe and Rupp (2013) suggest that the ACA may reduce disability lock for some people and allow them to return to work, which would reduce the number of people receiving disability benefits.

The ACA has the potential to affect disability insurance in ways not directly related to altering claiming incentives, such as through the ACA provisions that aim to reduce Medicare costs. These provisions, which were discussed in the second section of the chapter, directly affect SSDI beneficiaries, since Medicare is their health insurance. Many speculate that the IPAB may eventually cut Medicare reimbursement rates for doctors (Vaida 2012). While this would reduce costs to the Medicare program, it may also make it more difficult for SSDI recipients to receive medical care, since doctors may be less likely to accept Medicare patients. Cutting costs and improving care are goals of ACOs and reasons for not reimbursing preventable readmissions. Both these measures have the potential to decrease costs while improving the care that SSDI recipients receive.

In addition to decreasing the costs of applying for SSDI, improving health insurance options during the two-year waiting period may also increase the health care access of SSDI recipients. The two-year waiting period is often a concern, since SSDI recipients have health issues. Riley (2006) studies health insurance and health care access during the waiting period and finds that 26 percent of SSDI beneficiaries lacked health insurance during this period. He also finds that SSDI beneficiaries without health insurance had more problems accessing health care than those with health insurance. Weathers and Stegman (2012) and Michalopoulos et al. (2012) study a Social Security program that provides health insurance coverage to SSDI beneficiaries while they await Medicare eligibility. Weathers and Stegman find that these accelerated benefits increased mental health and physical health one year after enrollment. Although they find no evidence of changes in mortality, they point out that this increased health could lower costs once people are on SSDI. Michalopoulos et al. find that the accelerated benefits program resulted in people having fewer unmet medical needs and reduced out-of-pocket spending on medical care. They also find that accelerated benefits enrollees were more likely to search for work. These results indicate that the ACA may cause SSDI recipients to be healthier and more likely to exit disability.

By providing greater access to health care, the ACA may make it easier for people to obtain the documentation necessary to prove they have a disability. As part of the application for disability, applicants need to provide medical records about their disabilities, as well as contact information for all the relevant health care professionals, laboratory and test results, and the names of medicines they take (Social Security Administration 2014b). Making the documentation of a disability easier could result in more people applying for coverage or an increase in the acceptance rate among those who apply for benefits.

WORKERS' COMPENSATION

Basic Program Information

Workers' compensation pays all medical bills for individuals with work-related injuries and diseases. Unlike federal disability, workers' compensation is a state-level program. Therefore, all workers' compensation programs are a little different from each other. In some states, private insurance companies administer workers' compensation, while in others, the states are the sole providers of insurance. For workers who miss more than three to seven days of work, workers' compensation also replaces lost wages through indemnity benefits. The injured workers' weekly benefits are a function of their weekly earnings and are subject to state-level maximums. In all states except Texas and Oklahoma, workers' compensation insurance is mandatory for employers.

Injured workers receiving indemnity benefits usually first receive temporary total disability (TTD). They receive these benefits until they are able to return to work or are evaluated for permanent disability benefits. They will be evaluated for permanent disability benefits after they have reached the state limit for temporary benefits or the physician has determined they have reached "maximum medical improvement." Permanent disability benefits comprise two separate types of benefits: permanent total disability (PTD) and permanent partial disability (PPD). PTD and PPD benefits in that injured workers receive benefits based on their average weekly wages subject to the state maximum. Workers stop receiving benefits when they have healed, returned to work, or reached the state maximum number of weeks for PTD eligibility. With PPD benefits, workers are generally given a partial impairment rating or assigned a fixed schedule of benefits. People are typically allowed to work while receiving PPD benefits. (See McInerney and Simon [2012] for a more thorough discussion of different benefit types and Hunt [2004] for a discussion of the adequacy of those benefits.)

In 2011, nearly 126 million workers were covered by workers' compensation insurance (Sengupta, Baldwin, and Reno 2013). Employers paid over $77 billion for coverage, and workers received over $60 billion from the system. The majority of workers' compensation cases—around 76 percent—are medical-only cases and do not involve payments for missed work. Figure 5.3 shows workers' compensation spending on medical and wage replacement over time. Spending for wage replacement has been falling since the early 1990s, while medical spending has continued to rise. The share of medical benefits as a percentage of the total benefits paid for workers' compensation has risen from around 30 percent in the early 1980s to approximately 50 percent in 2011.

Figure 5.3 Workers' Compensation Medical and Indemnity Benefits by Year

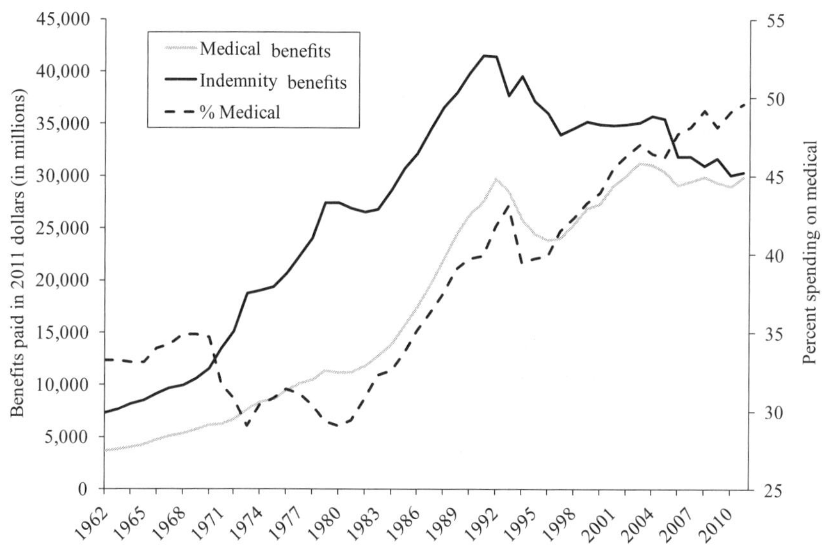

SOURCE: Sengupta, Baldwin, and Reno (2013).

The ACA's Potential Effect on Workers' Compensation

The ACA will change the incentive to claim workers' compensation by expanding health insurance coverage, which reduces the benefit of filing for workers' compensation, regardless of whether the injury is work related. People without health insurance have an increased incentive to claim that their medical issues are work related even if they are not so that workers' compensation will pay the bills. Thus, having health insurance may lower the incidence of people misclassifying non-work-related injuries. If an injury occurs at work, health insurance may still deter workers from filing a claim for workers' compensation if it is costly, and there are several reasons to believe that it is. First, employers may dissuade their employees from filing workers' compensation because they fear it will increase their premiums. Second, injured workers might not want to deal with the associated paperwork, or they may fear that they will be called on to prove that their injury was caused by work, which is not always easy to do. Filing with health insurance, meanwhile, requires no burden of proof. Third, there may be a stigma associated with filing a workers' compensation claim.

According to some studies, a large percentage of workers do not file a workers' compensation claim because they have health insurance. Biddle and Roberts (2003) surveyed Michigan workers identified by physicians as likely having work-related injuries. Of these injured workers, only 30 percent filed for workers' compensation. Of the 70 percent who did not file for workers' compensation, 36 percent said that having health insurance was the reason. However, Lakdawalla, Reville, and Seabury (2007) show that people with health insurance are generally more likely to receive workers' compensation. They hypothesize that large firms may be more likely to provide workers with information about workers' compensation and to encourage them to use it.

Heaton (2012) studies the impact of Massachusetts's health insurance reform on workers' compensation by projecting how many emergency room bills would have been paid for by the state's workers' compensation system in the absence of the 2006 reform based on 2005 Massachusetts data. Heaton finds that the health care reform resulted in workers' compensation paying for 5–10 percent fewer emergency room medical bills. He finds similarly sized decreases for both the overall patient population and those with relatively serious medical conditions.

In Dillender (2015a), using administrative medical claims data from Texas, I study the effect of health insurance on young adults filing workers' compensation claims. I compare individuals just before and after they turn 26, the age at which young adults lose access to dependent coverage under the ACA. This approach yields estimates of the causal effect of health insurance on workers' compensation filing. I find that immediately after people turn 26, initial claims filed for injuries with easy-to-delay reporting increase, while the overall amount of medical treatment that workers' compensation pays for increases by 8 percent. Despite these increases, overall workers' compensation medical costs do not increase dramatically for 26-year-olds because the majority of this increased care is for less expensive services. These results suggest that health insurance affects workers' compensation filing, particularly at the intensive margin, but not necessarily for the types of services that drive medical costs.

Overall, the empirical studies suggest that workers' compensation will pay for less medical care once more people have health insurance. In Dillender (2015a), I find evidence that the claiming behavior of people with minor medical needs is influenced by having health insurance. This would suggest that the overall savings to workers' compensation would be modest. Heaton (2012), however, finds evidence that people with greater medical needs respond to health reform, which suggests that the cost savings to workers' compensation could be large. Thus, while the evidence strongly suggests that the ACA will decrease the likelihood that health care is paid for by workers' compensation, the size of the cost savings to workers' compensation is difficult to assess. Also, if people with more severe medical issues respond to workers' compensation, indemnity claims may also respond by falling slightly as a result of the ACA; however, no research has explored if and how indemnity claims are affected by health insurance.

By influencing some people to file claims with health insurance instead of workers' compensation, the ACA may result in cost savings to the workers' compensation system. However, the ACA may also change the type of insurance plans people have by encouraging the use of more high-deductible plans—for example, with a 40 percent excise tax on health plans with individual premiums above $10,200 and family premiums above $27,500 starting in 2018 (Zuckerman 2010). Since people will lack first-dollar coverage, they may be more likely to shift claims onto workers' compensation, which will still provide first-dollar coverage.

The changes to Medicare discussed previously also have implications for workers' compensation, especially if the IPAB curtails Medicare costs by cutting reimbursement rates. Many states tie workers' compensation reimbursement rates to Medicare reimbursement rates. By cutting Medicare reimbursement rates, the ACA would also lower workers' compensation reimbursement rates in many states unless state governments react by changing their laws. Thus, the ACA will lower the amount of money spent on medical care. However, this may cause providers in these states to be less likely to accept workers' compensation patients since they will receive less money for treating them. Even in states that do not tie their reimbursement rates to Medicare, changes in Medicare rates may affect workers' compensation. Auerbach, Heaton, and Brantley (2014) argue that when Medicare pays physicians less, it may cause physicians to increase prices for other payers or provide more services to other patients that provide higher margins. If Medicare no longer pays providers for certain readmissions, it may have the same effect if it decreases physicians' profits from Medicare patients.

Auerbach, Heaton, and Brantley (2014) also argue that the ACA could change the composition of the labor force. A large literature in economics finds that the need for health insurance has induced people to participate in the labor force (Antwi, Moriya, and Simon 2013; Blau and Gilleskie 2001; Buchmueller and Carpenter 2012; Dillender 2015b; Nyce et al. 2013; Strumpf 2010). Prior to the ACA, there were few good health insurance options for the near elderly outside employment. Auerbach, Heaton, and Brantley argue that the exchanges and subsidies will allow older people to retire sooner, which may reduce costs, since older workers typically take longer to recover from injuries and require more treatment.

POTENTIAL EFFECTS OF THE ACA ON BOTH PROGRAMS

As both disability insurance and workers' compensation insurance tap into the same medical resources that health insurance does, they will both be affected by the aspects of the ACA that affect the medical system more generally. One potential impact of the ACA is to improve the health of the general population. Research typically finds that health insurance improves health (Card, Dobkin, and Maestas 2009; Doyle 2005; Finkelstein et al. 2012), and Courtemanche and Zapata (2014) find that people reported being in better health as a result of the Massachusetts reform. The ACA also has a focus on prevention by eliminating copayments for preventive services and including an annual wellness visit as a part of Medicare. This has the potential to lower the likelihood that people become disabled or suffer an injury while at work.

The ACA has various strategies to make medical treatment less expensive, such as with the Patient-Centered Outcomes Research Institute, which focuses on identifying effective treatments. The ACA also implements rules that establish electronic health records, which could also reduce costs while improving care. By identifying effective treatments and digitizing medical records, the ACA has the potential to lower costs for medical care paid under both disability insurance and workers' compensation.

A potential issue with the dramatic increase in insurance coverage promised by the ACA is that it will put more stress on existing medical resources. Hofer, Abraham, and Moscovice (2011) point out that there was already a shortage of primary care doctors before the ACA and suggest that the increased demand from the ACA could increase the shortages. Huang and Finegold (2013) find that certain areas will be hit hard by an increase in demand, while other areas will be able to meet the demand. They estimate that 7 million people live in areas where demand for primary care may exceed supply by 10 percent after the ACA. Physician shortages may increase wait times for injured and disabled people before they can receive medical care.

CONCLUSION

By overhauling the health insurance system and making many broad changes to medical care, the ACA promises to change the health care landscape. In this chapter, I describe the changes taking place because of the ACA, as well as their implications for two major social insurance programs with large medical components. I review the considerable evidence that suggests that expanding health insurance could affect claiming behavior for both disability and workers' compensation. For disability insurance, some evidence suggests that expanding health insurance may have countervailing effects on overall disability coverage. For workers' compensation, the evidence points to health insurance covering some of the costs that workers' compensation insurance was previously paying.

Apart from affecting claiming behavior, the ACA will likely affect these social insurance programs in other ways as well. The ACA's many cost-saving measures will likely have spillover effects for both disability insurance and workers' compensation, especially those measures that aim to identify the most effective treatments. The aspects of the ACA that aim to improve population health may also result in fewer work-related injuries and less disability, thereby saving money for both programs. One negative aspect of the ACA for both of these programs may be that the increase in insurance coverage puts more strain on medical resources, which could make seeing a doctor more difficult.

References

Antwi, Yaa Akosa, Asako S. Moriya, and Kosali Simon. 2013. "Effects of Federal Policy to Insure Young Adults: Evidence from the 2010 Affordable Care Act's Dependent-Coverage Mandate." *American Economic Journal: Economic Policy* 5(4): 1–28.

Auerbach, David I., Paul Heaton, and Ian Brantley. 2014. *How Will the Patient Protection and Affordable Care Act Affect Liability Insurance Costs?* Santa Monica, CA: RAND Corporation.

Autor, David H., and Mark G. Duggan. 2006. "The Growth in the Social Security Disability Rolls: A Fiscal Crisis Unfolding." *Journal of Economic Perspectives* 20(3): 71–96.

Biddle, Jeff, and Karen Roberts. 2003. "Claiming Behavior in Workers' Compensation." *Journal of Risk and Insurance* 70(4): 759–780.

Blau, David M., and Donna B. Gilleskie. 2001. "Retiree Health Insurance and the Labor Force Behavior of Older Men in the 1990s." *Review of Economics and Statistics* 83(1): 64–80.

Buchmueller, Thomas, and Christopher Carpenter. 2012. "The Effect of Requiring Private Employers to Extend Health Benefit Eligibility to Same-Sex Partners of Employees: Evidence from California." *Journal of Policy Analysis and Management* 31(2): 388–403.

Card, David, Carlos Dobkin, and Nicole Maestas. 2009. "Does Medicare Save Lives?" *Quarterly Journal of Economics* 124(2): 597–636.

Center on Budget and Policy Priorities. 2014. "Policy Basics: Introduction to Supplemental Security Income." Washington, DC: Center on Budget and Policy Priorities. http://www.cbpp.org/sites/default/files/atoms/files/PolicyBasics_SocSec-IntroToSSI.pdf (accessed September 4, 2015).

Coe, Norma, and Kalman Rupp. 2013. "Does Access to Health Insurance Influence Work Effort among Disability Cash Benefit Recipients?" Center for Retirement Research Working Paper 2013-10. Boston: Boston College, Center for Retirement Research.

Congressional Budget Office. 2014. "Updated Estimates of the Effects of the Insurance Coverage Provisions of the Affordable Care Act, April 2014." Washington, DC: Congressional Budget Office. http://www.cbo.gov/sites/default/files/cbofiles/attachments/45231-ACA_Estimates.pdf (accessed September 4, 2015).

Courtemanche, Charles J., and Daniela Zapata. 2014. "Does Universal Coverage Improve Health? The Massachusetts Experience." *Journal of Policy Analysis and Management* 33(1): 36–69.

Doyle, Joseph J. Jr. 2005. "Health Insurance, Treatment and Outcomes: Using Auto Accidents as Health Shocks." *Review of Economics and Statistics* 87(2): 256–270.

Dillender, Marcus. 2015a. "The Effect of Health Insurance on Workers' Compensation Filing: Evidence from the Affordable Care Act's Age-Based Threshold for Dependent Coverage." *Journal of Health Economics* 43: 204–228.

———. 2015b. "Health Insurance and Labor Force Participation: What Legal Recognition Does for Same-Sex Couples." *Contemporary Economic Policy* 33(2): 381–394.

Finkelstein, Amy, Sarah Taubman, Bill Wright, Mira Bernstein, Jonathan Gruber, Joseph P. Newhouse, Heidi Allen, and Katherine Baicker. 2012. "The Oregon Health Insurance Experiment: Evidence from the First Year." *Quarterly Journal of Economics* 127(3): 1057–1106.

Gruber, Jonathan, and Jeffrey Kubik. 2002. *Health Insurance Coverage and the Disability Insurance Application Decision*. NBER Working Paper No. 9148. Cambridge, MA: National Bureau of Economic Research.

Heaton, Paul. 2012. *The Impact of Health Care Reform on Workers' Compensation Medical Care*. RAND Institute for Civil Justice Technical Report. Santa Monica, CA: RAND Corporation.

Hill, Steven C. 2012. "Individual Insurance Benefits to Be Available under Health Reform Would Have Cut Out-of-Pocket Spending in 2001–08." *Health Affairs* 31(6): 1349–1356.

Hofer, Adam N., Jean Abraham, and Ira Moscovice. 2011. "Expansion of Coverage under the Patient Protection and Affordable Care Act and Primary Care Utilization." *Milbank Quarterly* 89(1): 69–89.

Huang, Elbert S., and Kenneth Finegold. 2013. "Seven Million Americans Live in Areas Where Demand for Primary Care May Exceed Supply by More than 10 percent." *Health Affairs* 32(3): 614–621.

Hunt, H. Allan, ed. 2004. *Adequacy of Earnings Replacement in Workers' Compensation Programs.* Washington, DC: National Academy of Social Insurance and Kalamazoo, MI: W. E. Upjohn Institute for Employment Research.

Kaiser Family Foundation. 2012. "A Guide to the Supreme Court's Decision on the ACA's Medicaid Expansion." Menlo Park, CA: Henry J. Kaiser Family Foundation.

———. 2013. "Summary of the Affordable Care Act." Last modified April 25, 2013. Menlo Park, CA: Henry J. Kaiser Family Foundation.

———. 2014. "Status of State Action on the Medicaid Expansion Decision, 2014." Menlo Park, CA: Henry J. Kaiser Family Foundation. http://kff.org/health-reform/state-indicator/state-activity-around-expanding-medicaid-under-the-affordable-care-act/ (accessed September 4, 2015).

Kolstad, Jonathan T., and Amanda E. Kowalski. 2012. "Mandate-Based Health Reform and the Labor Market: Evidence from the Massachusetts Reform." NBER Working Paper No. 17933. Cambridge, MA: National Bureau of Economic Research.

Lakdawalla, Darius N., Robert T. Reville, and Seth A. Seabury. 2007. "How Does Health Insurance Affect Workers' Compensation Filing?" *Economic Inquiry* 45(2): 286–303.

Maestas, Nicole, Kathleen Mullen, and Alexander Strand. 2014. "Disability Insurance and Health Insurance Reform: Evidence from Massachusetts." *American Economic Review:* (Papers and Proceedings) 104(5): 329–335.

McInerney, Melissa, and Kosali Simon. 2012. "The Effect of State Workers' Compensation Program Changes on the Use of Federal Social Security Disability Insurance." *Industrial Relations: A Journal of Economy and Society* 51(1): 57–88.

Michalopoulos, Charles, David Wittenburg, Dina A. R. Israel, and Anne Warren. 2012. "The Effects of Health Care Benefits on Health Care Use and Health: A Randomized Trial for Disability Insurance Beneficiaries." *Medical Care* 50(9): 764–771.

Moulta-Ali, Umar. 2013. "Primer on Disability Benefits: Social Security Disability Insurance (SSDI) and Supplemental Security Income (SSI)." Washington, DC: Congressional Research Service.

Nyce, Steven, Sylvester J. Schieber, John B. Shoven, Sita Nataraj Slavov, and

David A. Wise. 2013. "Does Retiree Health Insurance Encourage Early Retirement?" *Journal of Public Economics* 104: 40–51.

Riley, Gerald F. 2006. "Health Insurance and Access to Care among Social Security Disability Insurance Beneficiaries during the Medicare Waiting Period." *INQUIRY: The Journal of Health Care Organization, Provision, and Financing* 43(3): 222–230.

Schoen, Cathy, Michelle M. Doty, Ruth H. Robertson, and Sara R. Collins. 2011. "Affordable Care Act Reforms Could Reduce the Number of Underinsured U.S. Adults by 70 Percent." *Health Affairs* 30(9): 1762–1771.

Sengupta, Ishita, Marjorie Baldwin, and Virginia Reno. 2013. *Workers' Compensation: Benefits, Coverage, and Costs*. Washington, DC: National Academy of Social Insurance.

Social Security Administration. 2013. "Annual Statistical Supplement to the Social Security Bulletin, 2013." Washington, DC: Social Security Administration. http://www.ssa.gov/policy/docs/statcomps/supplement/2013/supplement13.pdf (accessed September 4, 2015).

———. 2014a. SSI Federal Payment Amounts. Washington, DC: Social Security Administration. http://www.ssa.gov/oact/cola/SSIamts.html (accessed September 4, 2015).

———. 2014b. "Social Security Disability Benefits." SSA Publication No. 05-10029. Washington, DC: Social Security Administration. http://www.socialsecurity.gov/pubs/EN-05-10029.pdf (accessed September 4, 2015).

———. 2014c. Statistical Tables. Washington, DC: Social Security Administration. http://www.ssa.gov/oact/STATS/index.html. http://www.socialsecurity.gov/OACT/STATS/ (accessed September 4, 2015).

———. 2014d. "2011 Annual Report of the SSI Program." Washington, DC: Social Security Administration. http://www.ssa.gov/oact/ssir/SSI11/Participants.html#646860 (accessed September 4, 2015).

Sommers, Benjamin D., Thomas Musco, Kenneth Finegold, Munira Z. Gunja, Amy Burke, and Audrey M. McDowell. 2014. "Health Reform and Changes in Health Insurance Coverage in 2014." *New England Journal of Medicine* 371(9): 867–874.

Strumpf, Erin. 2010. "Employer-Sponsored Health Insurance for Early Retirees: Impacts on Retirement, Health, and Health Care." *International Journal of Health Care Finance and Economics* 10(2): 105–147.

Vaida, Bara. 2012. "The IPAB: The Center of a Political Clash over How to Change Medicare." *Kaiser Health News*. Menlo Park, CA: Henry J. Kaiser Family Foundation. http://khn.org/news/ipab-faq (accessed September 4, 2015).

Weathers II, Robert R., and Michelle Stegman. 2012. "The Effect of Expanding Access to Health Insurance on the Health and Mortality of Social Security

Disability Insurance Beneficiaries." *Journal of Health Economics* 31(6): 863–875.

Zuckerman, Stephen. 2010. "What Are the Provisions in the New Law for Containing Costs and How Effective Will They Be?" Washington, DC: Urban Institute. http://www.urban.org/uploadedpdf/412194-ppaca-containing-costs.pdf (accessed September 4, 2015).

6
The Economic Challenges of the Community Living Assistance Services and Supports Act

Edward C. Norton
University of Michigan and National Bureau of Economic Research

The most controversial part of the Patient Protection and Affordable Care Act (ACA) is the mandate that individuals purchase health insurance. The individual mandate is justified on economic grounds to avoid an adverse selection death spiral in the individual health insurance market. The constitutionality of the individual mandate was challenged in court, with the plaintiffs arguing that the government could not compel individuals to participate in a market. However, the Supreme Court narrowly upheld the constitutionality of the individual mandate, allowing that part of the ACA to continue to be implemented gradually.

Lost from much of the public discourse about the ACA was that a major component of the original act—one that encouraged a special form of health insurance but not through a mandate—was dropped by the government and will not be implemented. The Community Living Assistance Services and Supports Act would have created a market for long-term care insurance, called the CLASS program. The goal was to provide assistance to working-age individuals who had difficulty performing daily activities and required long-term care services. The CLASS program was decidedly different from the ACA's approach to standard health insurance because it was to be voluntary and entirely self-financed; no one questioned its constitutionality. It was also extremely important politically in getting the entire ACA passed because it improved the Congressional Budget Office's (CBO) 10-year economic forecast for the entire act.

Despite the lack of controversy surrounding its constitutionality, the Senate Appropriations Committee eliminated funding for the design and marketing of the CLASS program in the fall of 2011 (Gleckman 2011). The Department of Health and Human Services (HHS) disbanded the CLASS program office, and the then-secretary Kathleen Sebelius stopped efforts to design the program. Congress has no plans to rescue it.

Why was the CLASS program dropped? What economic challenges did it face, given that it was not challenged on constitutional grounds? What is the proper role of government in providing an insurance market? This chapter addresses these questions.

BACKGROUND ISSUES

The greatest financial uncertainty for the elderly is not for food, pharmaceuticals, or even inpatient care, it is for long-term care (Norton, Wang, and Stearns 2006). The financial burden of long-term care (either nursing home care or home health care) can be large because insurance coverage is often modest, and because care can continue for a decade or more. Medicare insurance is quite complete for inpatient care, outpatient care, and pharmaceuticals, especially when considering Medigap and Medicaid policies that help with copayments and deductibles. But Medicare coverage of long-term care is quite limited and requires substantial cost sharing. This leaves long-term care as the greatest expenditure risk.

It is hard to predict years in advance who will need nursing home care. Some may die before they need care; others will lose their spouses, their health, and then their independence. When there is high financial risk and difficulty in predicting who will need benefits, there is an opportunity for private insurance.

Despite the apparent demand for long-term care insurance for the elderly, there are many reasons private long-term care insurance is seldom sold. This has been discussed extensively in the literature (see, e.g., Brown and Finkelstein [2007, 2011]; Frank [2012]; and Norton [2000]). Here is a brief summary of the most important reasons the private insurance market is small. Adverse selection means that those who are most likely to need long-term care are most likely to want to buy it; insurance companies may target individuals who statistically are least likely to need it. Moral hazard is also often a problem in insurance markets. For long-term care there is both standard moral hazard and a version proposed by Pauly (1990), in which elderly people do not buy insurance so that their children, the presumed future decision makers, will not put them in a nursing home. Loading (administrative) costs are high because most sales are made to individuals and because adverse selection requires background and health checks. Medicaid is a close substitute for part of the population who would qualify for Medicaid quickly. Insurance companies now offer capped daily benefits, instead of paying a fraction of the cost (like most other health insurance), because of the difficulty in predicting future nursing home costs (Cutler 1996). This reduces the insurance value of the product and lowers its desirability. Some elderly people greatly underestimate their own risk of needing long-term care, again lowering demand (Frank 2012). Given all these reasons combined, it is perhaps a wonder anyone buys long-term care insurance.

The target population for the CLASS program was working-age adults who face a small risk of disability during their working years. This population is younger on average than those who first consider purchasing long-term care insurance. While the specifics of financial uncertainty and lack of insurance are slightly different than for the older population insuring against the need for nursing home care, the main themes apply to this younger population. If someone becomes disabled to a degree that they cannot work or live independently, then she faces enormous financial risks. Having a steady supply of cash could make the difference between remaining independent at home and going to an institution, but currently there is not an adequate private market for this. Presumably, the same issues of adverse selection, moral hazard, loading, competition from close substitutes, and misperceptions also apply.

An alternative to formal long-term care (nursing home and home health care) is informal care, unpaid care that is typically provided by close relatives (Grabowski, Norton, and Van Houtven 2012). Studies have shown that receiving informal care can reduce formal home health and nursing home use and cost (Van Houtven and Norton 2004, 2008). Informal caregivers may not only help keep loved ones out of nursing homes, they also may enjoy time with their relatives and set a good example for the next generation. However, there can be costs too. The caregiver may need to quit his job or work reduced hours, and the caregiver's own health may suffer during the course of helping others (Coe and Van Houtven 2009; Do et al. 2014).

When there is no private market for something that some people clearly desire, there may be room for the government to step in and create a market. Justification would depend on whether the government can overcome existing market failures. Given this background, there is clearly room for discussion about the possible role of government in creating a market for long-term care insurance.

THE CLASS ACT

The CLASS Act was Title VIII of the ACA. The purpose was to provide a cash benefit for nonmedical care and for support to help people live in the community. The cash benefit could have been used to purchase home health care, to reimburse relatives for their time, or to purchase other support. One goal was to keep people out of expensive nursing homes and thereby keep them in their homes, where they are generally happier. Another goal was to reduce government expenditures on long-term care. For critical summaries of the CLASS Act, see Miller (2011) and Wiener (2012).

The CLASS program was one form of consumer-directed long-term care services and was related to the policy of cash and counseling, which provides both cash to needy elderly persons with no strings attached and also counseling about effective ways to spend the cash. Again, the goals of cash and counseling programs were to keep people in their homes and lower the cost of long-term care. Cash and counseling demonstration programs in three states began in 1998 (Doty, Mahoney, and Sciegaj 2010) and are now used in several states (San Antonio et al. 2010; Simon-Rusinowitz et al. 2010) and in several other countries (Low et al. 2012; Nadash et al. 2012).

The two key features of the CLASS program were in stark contrast to the standard health insurance policy in the ACA: it was voluntary and self-financed. Because no one would have been compelled to buy it, there was no debate over the constitutionality of the policy. Of course, this was potentially a great weakness of the CLASS Act—if not enough healthy people signed up for it, it would not have been financially sustainable.

Being self-financed, the CLASS program would not have been subsidized from general tax revenues; all benefits would have been paid from premiums. Furthermore, the program was required to be financially sustainable for at least 75 years. This politically important requirement imposed tough conditions on running the program. Long-run financial solvency is hard to maintain, as will be discussed below.

There were several other important provisions about benefits in the CLASS Act. Premiums were to be used for consumer-directed services, meaning that the consumer would decide how to spend the money, similar to cash and counseling programs. For example, the money could have been used to pay for informal care by a son or daughter. The benefit, by statute, had to be at least $50 per day, but it could also have been adjusted by the level of disability. There were no lifetime limits on benefits. Additional benefits included advocacy and financial advice.

The CLASS program insurance had no underwriting, meaning that premiums were not adjusted for risk, such as for health status or chronic conditions; all persons of the same age paid the same premium. A healthy person in a low-risk job would pay the same premium as a chronically disabled person who is waiting for the end of the vesting period to start collecting benefits. Therefore, the actuarial value of the insurance is high for a person with a high risk of needing the insurance, and low for a person with low risk. The low actuarial value for persons with low risk contributes greatly to the problem of adverse selection because demand for such insurance depends on the actuarial value of what is being purchased.

Eligibility for receiving benefits from the CLASS Act had two conditions, beyond signing up and paying premiums. First, a person would have to pay into the system for at least five years before being eligible to receive any benefits. This was an extraordinarily long vesting period for individual insurance and was necessary because of concerns about adverse selection. The other condition for eligibility is that during the vesting period the person had to be working. However, the definition of working had a low bar—annual earnings of at least $1,200. Even working at minimum wage, it would take fewer than four hours per week to earn the minimum.

Despite the length of the written legislation, the ACA left many important details to be worked out after passage. The HHS secretary was charged with determining many specific details within the broad parameters outlined in the ACA. For example, eligibility was to be determined primarily by disability level, but the details of what that level would be (such as activities of daily living or mental health) were up to the secretary. Eligibility could have also potentially changed if the person did in fact enter a nursing home or hospital or become Medicaid eligible. For example, if the one goal of the CLASS Act were to reduce admissions to nursing homes, why should someone receive the cash benefit after admission? By law, the benefit level needed to be at least $50 per day. The cash benefits could have been adjusted for the level of disability. Also unspecified was whether there would be differences by financial need at the time, by family status or geographic location. Although the premiums were not allowed to be risk adjusted, it was left open whether premiums would be adjusted for income (or wealth), student status, or marital status. The big unknown was the price elasticity for premiums—if it was high, then small increases in the premium would have large detrimental effects on enrollment, revenues, and long-run financial stability.

Had the CLASS Act been implemented, it would have been rolled out on a timetable roughly similar to the rest of the ACA. The HHS secretary was due to release rules for eligibility and enrollment in January 2012. By October 2012 the secretary was to announce benefit design and premiums. People could have begun purchasing insurance by 2014. However, in the fall of 2011, the secretary announced that the CLASS program would not be implemented (Gleckman 2011).

The Congressional Budget Office (CBO) scores every proposed piece of legislation over a 10-year horizon to see what the net financial effect will be on the national budget. A positive score means that the legislation will save more money than it will spend. Because of proposed expansions to Medicaid and subsidies to purchase individual health insurance, there was concern that the overall score for the ACA would be negative. The CLASS Act was existing legislation that could be added to the rest of the ACA. Most importantly, it was sure to have a positive score over a 10-year period. The act's five-year vesting period ensures that people pay in for many years before receiving benefits. So, over a 10-year horizon (especially with a few years of start up at the beginning), the CLASS Act was sure to improve the overall CBO score. This is one way that the act became important politically in the development of the ACA.

The CBO had to make reasonable assumptions about how the program would be run, such as that the average monthly premium would be $123 and that the average daily benefit would be $75. It assumed modest reductions in Medicaid payments on long-term care, and also that the program would remain solvent over a 75-year period. With those assumptions, the CBO estimated that the CLASS Act alone would reduce the federal deficit by $74 billion over 10 years. This was roughly half of the total projected savings of $138 billion for the entire ACA.

ECONOMIC PROBLEMS

The CLASS program faced formidable economic challenges. The goal was to create an insurance product that provided needed services to the general public while also remaining financially viable in the long run. The legislation set certain parameters—particularly on benefits, eligibility, and underwriting—that made it impossible to succeed. In this section I review the economic challenges with designing such a system and why the program was doomed to fail.

The first question is, why should the government be involved in this market at all? Why not leave it to the private sector? If it were possible to sell an insurance product to the general population and make money (the basic terms and conditions of the CLASS Act), the private market would figure out how to do it. And if the private market cannot sell an insurance product at a profit under these terms, the government would need to think hard about whether a public solution could work when a private solution cannot.

There is a modest-sized private market for long-term care insurance, but it is now shrinking. To be clear, this private market is aimed at providing insurance for the elderly against the risk of paying for nursing home care and home health care. This risk grows rapidly after age 70. The CLASS Act, in contrast, aims to provide services for working-age adults who become disabled, although the benefits could continue into old age. Therefore, while most of the issues are similar, the target audience for typical private long-term care insurance is slightly different than for the CLASS program.

Given the large and variable out-of-pocket expenditure risk faced by working-age adults, why is the private market so small? There are many reasons why insurance markets can fail. I review in more detail the list of reasons for the failure of the long-term care insurance market discussed before, and I further explore to what extent these reasons apply to the CLASS program. The two general problems for nearly all insurance markets are adverse selection and moral hazard. Adverse selection is a problem for private long-term care insurance if the bad risks are more likely to try to purchase insurance. An individual is likely to know more about her own health and health behaviors than the insurance company, such as risk of injury at work, family medical history (how long did her parents and other relatives live, and what were the causes of death?), household income and wealth, and family relationships (would a daughter be likely to provide informal care?). Adverse selection problems are mitigated somewhat by the long time horizon (what will happen to health, behaviors, and family status in 30 years?) and by the fact that, given demographics, the insurance company knows the actuarial risks extremely well. "Moral hazard" refers to a change in behavior after a person purchases insurance because the price of care is lower for an insured person. Unlike insurance for nursing home care, where few people desire to live in such a facility, for the working-age population cash benefits have high value.

For the CLASS program market, both adverse selection and moral hazard were likely to be even bigger problems than for the elderly long-term care insurance market. Any working-age adult with a chronic disability would have immediately signed up for the program. This problem was clearly foremost in the minds of the legislators who drafted this legislation because of the five-year vesting period, an astonishingly long time for any form of insurance. Moral hazard would also be a big problem because the benefit could be used in a wide variety of ways, including giving the cash to family members. Who would not want such a benefit?

There are cases where private markets break down, leaving a role for government intervention (Norton and Newhouse 1994). In such cases, government policy may have had the ability to surmount these problems in a way that the private market cannot. For example, one way to overcome moral hazard is to require broad participation. The ACA mandates insurance purchase (or a fine) to ensure broad participation of all, including the healthy, thereby combating adverse selection. However, participation was strictly voluntary for the CLASS program. Therefore, the government did not use any coercive means to combat adverse selection and relied instead on marketing campaigns to encourage enrollment by the relatively young and healthy. The restriction on underwriting makes adverse selection even worse. By not pricing the insurance to reflect expected costs (other than age), it is then relatively inexpensive for those chronically ill and relatively expensive for those who are healthy. This pricing encourages purchase by those most likely to use it and discourages purchase by those least likely to use it. There is a reason that insurance companies want to adjust premiums to reflect expected costs. When that pricing strategy is not allowed, it encourages adverse selection and will quickly undermine the financial viability of the insurance.

One way that the CLASS program would probably have had a competitive edge over private market rivals is through loading, or administrative overhead, which adds to the premium and makes the insurance attractive only to those who are quite risk averse. The load for private long-term care insurance has been estimated to be about 32 percent (Brown and Finkelstein 2011). It is high because it is mostly sold to individuals, with brokers receiving high commission fees. The government presumably could have sold the insurance with lower overhead, which lowers the premium and raises the value of the insurance, thereby increasing demand.

An additional challenge to the CLASS Act insurance was that it would have competed with a variety of products that are partial substitutes. Social Security pays disability benefits to people who have worked but now have a medical condition expected to last at least a year. Worker's compensation pays benefits to workers injured on the job. Medicaid provides both health insurance and long-term care insurance to people who meet their state's eligibility requirements, and those can include working-age adults with disabilities who have low incomes. And many people who need care assume (often correctly) that they can rely on their spouse, family, or extended family to provide long-term care services if they are ever needed. Alternative forms of insurance lower the demand for another substitute insurance product.

The long time span from initial purchase to ultimate use of benefits causes several problems for this insurance market. One of these is nondiversifiable intertemporal risk (Cutler 1996; Norton 2000). Long-term care insurance is usually for the future, not the upcoming year, as with regular health insurance. There are two big unknowns about expenditure risk in, say, 30 years: probability of use and price. The risk of probability of use can be diversified over a large general population. The price risk (what will the cost of home health care be in 30 years?) cannot be diversified across the population; large price increases affect everyone. Insurance companies do not like to take on nondiversifiable risk. Several decades ago, long-term care insurance companies switched from paying a percentage of fees (like most regular health insurance) to paying a flat daily fee. The capitated per diem limits the insurance company's exposure to the risk of price inflation. However, it also greatly reduces the value of purchasing insurance and hence lowers demand. The CLASS Act offers a capitated per diem benefit (perhaps adjusted for disability level). This means that the insurance protects against the extensive margin of any use but not the risk of intensive margin of the amount of use. That is, if the benefit is $50 per day and you need $200 to live independently, you are not protected for the extra $150.

Another problem with the long time horizon is that over an extended period, some people may lapse their premium payments. This could be due to the loss of the means to pay, a change in mind about the value of continuing to purchase the insurance, or simple forgetfulness. For private long-term care insurance, lapse in payment is a wonderful thing. When someone lapses, they forfeit past payments, which become pure profits to the company. Lapsed policies have been an important part of the business model of selling long-term care insurance. When a policy lapses, then the individual has to start over, like a new customer, at a higher price appropriate for her current age. In fact, one reason many insurance companies are no longer selling new long-term care insurance policies is that the lapse rates have declined, squeezing margins. Politically, the federal government could not encourage lapses as a way to keep the CLASS program solvent. The CLASS Act had a provision to allow a person to reenroll at a higher premium after lapsing, but there was a tricky balance. Minimizing lapses reduces financial viability. Also, if the policy on lapses is too weak, allowing people to skip payments during down times, there is the possibility for abuse.

To be successful, the CLASS program would have needed many healthy low-risk people to enroll. One way to increase enrollment would have been to encourage employers to offer the insurance as part of the benefit package. Getting the word out through large employers, and having people make decisions about the CLASS program at the same time as other benefit decisions, would undoubtedly increase enrollment. Another way to increase enrollment through employers would have been to offer it as an opt-out benefit. That is, the default would be to have employees signed up, although an employee could opt out by actively making a choice. Studies of benefit choice have shown that employees tend to go with default choices and tend to stick with past choices (Madrian and Shea 2001). An opt-out system offered through employers would dramatically increase enrollment; however, it is not clear whether employers would want to encourage employees to take up this insurance.

The legal status of premiums paid by the employee and collected by the employer complicates employers' ability to offer CLASS program insurance. Legally, if an employee has Social Security and other federal benefits deducted from their paychecks, then they get credit for having paid them; the employer is responsible for turning the premiums over to the IRS. If the employer is negligent in paying the IRS, then the employee is not held responsible. However, the legal status of the CLASS program premiums was different. Unless the IRS modified its rules, an employer could have collected premiums for the CLASS program and not turned them over, and the employee would be held responsible. Presumably the IRS could have amended its policies, but that did not happen.

Finally, there was the big unanswered question about what would happen if, down the road, the CLASS Act was later declared financially unstable. Suppose, for example, that the CLASS Act went into effect, and for its first 20 years was deemed financially solvent in the long run. But then, for some unfixable reason in the twenty-first year it was no longer financially solvent over the 75-year time horizon, as required by Congress. What would happen to everyone's premiums? Would people get them back? Would they get them back with interest? Forfeit everything? I asked several policymakers that question and never got an answer. No one wanted to talk about that possibility. Yet, I think the lack of an answer was important in undermining the financial feasibility of the CLASS Act. Why should I invest in something that is known to be financially risky if I do not know what will happen to my investment? If the CLASS Act promised to reimburse all enrollees, it would make the initial investment in the insurance more financially attractive.

CONCLUSION

In summary, the CLASS Act offered an insurance policy that was extremely expensive for relatively healthy people and thereby discouraged enrollment due to adverse selection. It did not protect against one major form of risk (risk of future price inflation), and it was unclear what would happen to paid premiums if the program were to be declared financially unstable in the long run. Having lower loading would not make up for the other fiscal problems. Given the constraints, the CLASS Act could never be financially solvent or fiscally responsible.

References

Brown, Jeffrey R., and Amy Finkelstein. 2007. "Why Is the Market for Long-Term Care Insurance So Small?" *Journal of Public Economics* 91(10): 1967–1991.

———. 2011. "Insuring Long-Term Care in the United States." *Journal of Economic Perspectives* 25(4): 119–141.

Coe, Norma B., and Courtney H. Van Houtven. 2009. "Caring for Mom and Neglecting Yourself? The Health Effects of Caring for an Elderly Parent." *Health Economics* 18(9): 991–1010.

Cutler, David M. 1996. "Why Don't Markets Insure Long-Term Risk?" Cambridge, MA: Harvard University and National Bureau of Economic Research.

Do, Young Kyung, Edward C. Norton, Sally C. Stearns, and Courtney H. Van Houtven. 2014. "Informal Care and Caregiver's Health." *Health Economics* 23(9): 993–1006.

Doty, Pamela, Kevin J. Mahoney, and Mark Sciegaj. 2010. "New State Strategies to Meet Long-Term Care Needs." *Health Affairs* 29(1): 49–56.

Frank, Richard G. 2012. "Long-Term Care Financing in the United States: Sources and Institutions." *Applied Economic Perspectives and Policy* 34(2): 333–345.

Gleckman, Howard. 2011. "Requiem for the CLASS Act." *Health Affairs* 30(12): 2231–2234.

Grabowski, David C., Edward C. Norton, and Courtney H. Van Houtven. 2012. "Informal Care." In *The Elgar Companion to Health Economics, Second Edition*, Andrew M. Jones, ed. Northampton, MA: Edward Elgar, pp. 318–328.

Low, Lee-Fay, Natalie Chilko, Meredith Gresham, Sarah Barter, and Henry Brodaty. 2012. "An Update on the Pilot Trial of Consumer-Directed Care for Older Persons in Australia." *Australasian Journal on Ageing* 31(1): 47–51.

Madrian, Brigitte C., and Dennis F. Shea. 2001. "The Power of Suggestion: Inertia in 401(k) Participation and Savings Behavior." *Quarterly Journal of Economics* 116(4): 1149–1187.

Miller, Edward Alan. 2011. "Flying Beneath the Radar of Health Reform: The Community Living Assistance Services and Supports (CLASS) Act." *Gerontologist* 51(2): 145–155.

Nadash, Pamela, Pamela Doty, Kevin J. Mahoney, and Matthias Von Schwanenflugel. 2012. "European Long-Term Care Programs: Lessons for Community Living Assistance Services and Supports?" *Health Services Research* 47(1): 309–328.

Norton, Edward C. 2000. "Long-Term Care." In *Handbook of Health Economics*, Vol. IB, Anthony J. Culyer and Joseph P. Newhouse, eds. New York: Elsevier Science B.V., pp. 956–994.

Norton, Edward C., and Joseph P. Newhouse. 1994. "Policy Options for Public Long-Term Care Insurance." *Journal of the American Medical Association* 271(19): 1520–1524.

Norton, Edward C., Hua Wang, and Sally C. Stearns. 2006. "Behavioral Implications of Out-of-Pocket Health Care Expenditures." *Swiss Journal of Economics and Statistics* 142(Special Issue): 3–11.

Pauly, Mark V. 1990. "The Rational Nonpurchase of Long-Term-Care Insurance." *Journal of Political Economy* 98(1): 153–168.

San Antonio, Patricia, Lori Simon-Rusinowitz, Dawn Loughlin, J. Kevin Eckert, Kevin J. Mahoney, and Kathleen Ann Depretis Ruben. 2010. "Lessons from the Arkansas Cash and Counseling Program: How the Experiences of Diverse Older Consumers and Their Caregivers Address Family Policy Concerns." *Journal of Aging & Social Policy* 22(1): 1–17.

Simon-Rusinowitz, Lori, Genevieve Martinez Garcia, Dana Martin, Michele Debarthe Sadler, Jane Tilly, Lori N. Marks, Dawn M. Loughlin, and Kevin J. Mahoney. 2010. "Hiring Relatives as Caregivers in Two States: Developing an Education and Research Agenda for Policy Makers." *Social Work in Public Health* 25(1): 17–41.

Van Houtven, Courtney H., and Edward C. Norton. 2004. "Informal Care and Health Care Use of Older Adults." *Journal of Health Economics* 23(6):1159–1180.

———. 2008. "Informal Care and Medicare Expenditures: Testing for Heterogeneous Treatment Effects." *Journal of Health Economics* 27(1): 134–156.

Wiener, Joshua M. 2012. "The CLASS Act: Is It Dead or Just Sleeping?" *Journal of Aging & Social Policy* 24(2): 118–135.

7
The Role of Private Health Insurance in the Medicare Program

M. Kate Bundorf
Stanford University

Medicare, the federal program that provides health insurance for aged and disabled people, is popular in the United States. While the majority of Americans report that they prefer spending cuts to higher taxes to reduce the government deficit, fewer than one in five support major reductions to Medicare (Kaiser Family Foundation 2011). But Medicare is expensive. In 2012, program expenditures totaled $574 billion—over $12,000 for each person enrolled (Lew et al. 2013). Medicare spending as a share of gross domestic product (GDP) is forecasted to increase from 3.6 percent in 2012 to 5.8 percent by 2035 as growth in Medicare spending continues to outpace growth in GDP. Between 2008 and 2012, approximately half of the growth in Medicare spending was driven by increasing utilization per beneficiary, and half was driven by rising enrollment due to the aging of the population (Chandra, Holmes, and Skinner 2013).

Devoting a greater share of resources to health care is not in itself necessarily problematic. Most economists believe that technological change has been the key driver of the persistent rise in health care spending both in the United States and in other countries (Fuchs 1996), and technological innovation in areas such as cardiovascular care, neonatal intensive care, and the treatment of mental health conditions has dramatically improved health and well-being for many (Cutler 2004). In other words, health care spending is often "worth it" in the sense that the benefits we gain from health care services exceed their cost. Higher spending on health care is also a natural consequence of rising income. As people become wealthier, they devote a greater share of their incomes to health care as the incremental value they receive from other types of consumption declines (Hall and Jones 2007).

In the context of the Medicare program, however, current spending levels are problematic for two reasons. First, Medicare is financed primarily through taxes, and program spending is a key driver of the $1.2 trillion U.S. federal budget deficit. Between 1973 and 2012, the percentage of the federal budget devoted to Medicare increased from 3.7 percent to 15.6 percent, and Medicare, Medicaid, and Social Security account for the vast majority of the projected growth of federal spending over the next decade (Congressional Budget Office 2013).

A more fundamental issue, however, is whether the current amount spent on Medicare produces enough value. A large body of literature documenting differences across geographic areas in the use of Medicare-financed services points to substantial inefficiency in the delivery of Medicare-financed services (Institute of Medicine 2013). Area-level spending differences do not appear to be explained by differences in health status of beneficiaries (Fisher et al. 2003; MedPAC 2011), and beneficiaries in high-use areas do not appear to be more satisfied with their care or have better patient outcomes (Baicker and Chandra 2004; Fisher et al. 2003; Skinner, Staiger, and Fisher 2006). Based on these types of studies, researchers have estimated that 20–30 percent of Medicare spending provides little to no improvement in health (Institute of Medicine 2011). In short, not only does there exist enormous opportunity to provide Medicare-financed services more efficiently, but reducing the rate of growth of Medicare spending is essential for fiscal stability.

Very few Medicare beneficiaries rely solely on the traditional Medicare program for insurance coverage. Because Medicare has relatively high deductibles and cost sharing for covered services and does not include long-term or dental care, most beneficiaries supplement their Medicare coverage with additional private or public insurance. State Medicaid programs provide publicly financed supplemental coverage for approximately 20 percent of beneficiaries with low incomes and modest assets, and approximately 30 percent of beneficiaries receive supplemental insurance from a former employer, although employer-sponsored retiree coverage is expected to decline dramatically since the number of employers offering retiree health insurance to current workers has declined sharply in recent years (Kaiser Family Foundation 2012).

Those without coverage from either Medicaid or former employers rely on highly regulated private insurance markets. Medicare Part C, or Medicare Advantage (MA), is a voluntary, private replacement for traditional Medicare, whereas Medigap is a private, individual policy that supplements Medicare. These two systems—private insurance supplementing and private insurance replacing a publicly funded benefit—represent alternative models for how public and private insurance interact. This chapter examines these different approaches and identifies the implications for Medicare reform.

MEDICARE: THE BASICS

Medicare provides health insurance for adults aged 65 and over and for younger people with disabilities, permanent kidney failure (end-stage renal disease), or amyotrophic lateral sclerosis (Lou Gehrig's disease). In 2012, Medicare covered 60 percent of the population—42.1 million aged 65 or older and 8.5 million disabled—and program expenditures totaled $574.2 billion (22 percent of national health spending) (Kaiser Family Foundation 2012; Lew et al. 2013). Prior to Medicare's establishment in 1965, roughly half of older adults in the United States had health insurance; now, nearly all have coverage (Moon 1996). The federal program is funded primarily through taxes and is administered by the Centers for Medicaid and Medicare Services (CMS), which functions as a public insurer, paying for services from private providers on behalf of Medicare beneficiaries. In 2012, Medicare covered 16 percent of the population and financed 22 percent of national health spending.

Medicare is technically composed of four distinct parts, referred to as parts A–D. Parts A and B, which were established when Medicare was enacted in 1965, were modeled after the typical types of insurance coverage available in the private market at the time. Part A, the Hospital Insurance program, covers inpatient hospital services, skilled nursing facilities, hospice care, and some home health care. In 2013, Medicare beneficiaries paid a deductible of $1,184 for the first 60 days in the hospital and $296 per day in coinsurance for days 61–90. For years in which beneficiaries use more than 90 inpatient days, they have 60 "lifetime reserve days" with coinsurance of $592 per day. After the reserve days are used, beneficiaries pay all costs of additional hospital inpatient care. Part B, part of the Supplementary Medical Insurance program, covers physician, outpatient, home health, and preventive services. In 2013, the deductible for Part B services was $147, and beneficiaries paid 20 percent of the Medicare-approved amount for most physician services.

Part A is funded by a payroll tax, and most people do not pay a premium when they enroll. Part B, in contrast, is funded by general tax revenues and beneficiary premiums. The monthly premium in 2013 was $104.90 for most beneficiaries but was higher for beneficiaries with incomes exceeding $85,000 for those filing individual income tax returns and $170,000 for those filing jointly. The vast majority of people who enroll in Part A also enroll in Part B, likely because the value to the beneficiary of the benefits is high relative to the cost and because the process of enrolling is administratively straightforward (Remler and Glied 2003). In this chapter, we refer to the combination of Parts A and B as "traditional Medicare."

Part C, also known as the Medicare Advantage program (MA), allows beneficiaries to enroll in a private health insurance plan as an alternative to the traditional Part A and Part B benefits. A participating private plan agrees to provide Medicare-covered services for beneficiaries and receives a payment from Medicare on behalf of each enrollee.

Part D, a highly subsidized outpatient prescription drug benefit, was established by the Medicare Modernization Act of 2003. The benefit is delivered exclusively by private insurers, and beneficiaries must actively enroll in a private plan in order to obtain coverage. Insurers may offer Part D benefits as stand-alone plans or as part of an MA plan. Part D plans also charge beneficiaries premiums for enrolling, and the premiums vary across plans. Enrollee premiums are waived, however, for very low-income beneficiaries, and higher-income beneficiaries must pay an additional monthly premium. Although Part D is clearly an important component of Medicare coverage, in this chapter we focus on Parts A and B, which provide medical as opposed to pharmaceutical coverage.

MEDICARE AND PRIVATE HEALTH INSURANCE

Traditional Medicare coverage, the combination of Parts A and B, is characterized by broad access to health care providers and relatively high cost sharing. Most health care providers participate in Medicare, and beneficiaries with Parts A and B are free to seek care from any physician, in contrast to most private plans serving the under-65 market, which restrict coverage to a limited set of providers. Due to its relatively high cost sharing, however, the Medicare basic benefit is substantively less generous than typical employer-sponsored coverage, and the cap on benefits for inpatient care exposes beneficiaries to significant financial risk (MedPAC 2011). On average, Medicare covers 64 percent of beneficiary spending on health care services for noninstitutionalized beneficiaries, and annual out-of-pocket liabilities average over $15,000 for the top 2 percent of spenders (MedPAC 2011).

Relatively few beneficiaries, however, are exposed to the cost-sharing provisions of the basic benefit, since most have supplemental insurance. The Medicare program offers two models of how private insurance interacts with publicly funded coverage: insurance supplementing publicly funded coverage (Medigap) and insurance replacing publicly funded coverage (MA). For both types of coverage, private plans compete for enrollees in markets highly regulated at the federal level.

Medigap

A market for private insurance supplementing Medicare quickly emerged after the introduction of Medicare in 1965, and state regulation soon followed in response to marketing abuses by some insurers and concerns over the ability of Medicare beneficiaries to make informed decisions about private coverage (Cafferata 1985). Many states introduced laws requiring minimum standards for nongroup Medigap policies in the 1970s, and in 1980 Congress passed legislation encouraging greater state-level regulation through a system of voluntary certification of Medicare supplemental policies (Government Accountability Office 1986; McCall, Rice, and Hall 1987; McCall, Rice, and Sangl 1986).

The Omnibus Reconciliation Act of 1990, which shifted much of the responsibility for regulation of the Medigap market from the state to the federal level and made requirements mandatory rather than voluntary, created the basic regulatory framework under which the market currently operates (Fox, Rice, and Alecxih 1995). The act mandated standardized benefits by restricting the sale of insurance supplementing Medicare to a set of 10 predefined plans, identified as plans A–J, and created a six-month open enrollment period for 65-year-olds newly entering the program, requiring guaranteed issue and prohibiting the use of health information in rate setting during this period (McCormack et al. 1996). The set of standardized plans that insurers are allowed to offer has changed somewhat over time, and, with the introduction of Medicare Part D, plans covering prescription drugs are no longer sold.

Medigap insurance helps beneficiaries pay for some of the health care costs that traditional Medicare does not cover. Table 7.1 describes the types of Medigap plans that insurers are permitted to sell. The plans cover primarily the coinsurance and deductibles associated with Parts A and B. In particular, all plans are required to cover Part A coinsurance, as well as up to 365 additional hospital days after Medicare-covered hospital days have been used. All plans also cover either all or some of the coinsurance or copayments for Medicare Part B services. The most popular plans, C and F, also cover the Part A and Part B deductibles.

Medicare Advantage

The main alternative to Medigap insurance is a Part C private plan (Medicare Advantage). The Medicare Advantage program was established by the Tax Equity and Fiscal Responsibility Act of 1982 and aimed to both expand the types of coverage available to Medicare beneficiaries and lower Medicare spending (McGuire, Newhouse, and Sinaiko 2011). The act authorized Medicare to contract with private plans to provide Medicare-covered services for beneficiaries and allowed Medicare enrollees to replace traditional Medicare with coverage from a qualified private plan. Participating plans sign an annual contract with the CMS, agreeing to provide benefits to beneficiaries and receive a capitated payment from the CMS for each beneficiary who enrolls. Historically, the CMS linked plan payments to the level of Medicare spending among fee-for-service enrollees in a geographic area, setting payments at 95 percent of the adjusted average per capita

Table 7.1 Medigap Plans

Medigap benefits (%)	A	B	C	D	F[a]	G	K[b]	L[b]	M	N[c]
Medicare Part A coinsurance and hospital costs up to an additional 365 days after Medicare benefits are used up	100	100	100	100	100	100	100	100	100	100
Medicare Part B coinsurance or copayment	100	100	100	100	100	100	50	75	100	100[c]
Blood (first 3 pints)	100	100	100	100	100	100	50	75	100	100
Part A hospice care coinsurance or copayment	100	100	100	100	100	100	50	75	100	100
Skilled nursing facility care coinsurance			100	100	100	100	50	75	100	100
Medicare Part A deductible		100	100	100	100	100	50	75	50	100
Medicare Part B deductible			100		100					
Medicare Part B excess charges					100	100				
Foreign travel emergency (up to plan limits)			100	100	100	100			100	100

[a] Plan F also offers a high-deductible plan. If you choose this option, you must pay for Medicare-covered costs up to the deductible amount of $2,110 in 2013 before your Medigap plan pays anything.

[b] For Plans K and L, after you meet your out-of-pocket yearly limit and your yearly Part B deductible ($147 in 2013), the Medigap plan pays 100% of covered services for the rest of the calendar year. The out-of-pocket limit for Plan K is $4,800; for Plan L it is $2,400.

[c] Plan N pays 100% of the Part B coinsurance, except for a copayment of up to $20 for some office visits and up to a $50 copayment for emergency room visits that don't result in an inpatient admission.

cost in the county and adjusting the payment for each enrollee for certain demographic characteristics (Pope et al. 2004).

Plans must provide a minimum level of benefits equivalent to that of Medicare and often provide additional benefits, such as lower cost sharing and additional covered services. As in the under 65 market, most MA plans contract with a limited set of providers in a given area. Thus, when choosing between the traditional Medicare program and an MA plan, beneficiaries are generally exchanging lower cost sharing for restrictions on provider access. While plans may charge beneficiaries a premium for enrolling, within a given service area, the premium must not vary by beneficiary characteristics.

The Balanced Budget Act of 1997 and subsequent legislation made a variety of changes to the program, including allowing types of plans other than HMOs to participate, changing the plan payment formula to encourage plans to enter in historically low-payment geographic areas, and requiring the CMS to improve its risk-adjustment methods (McGuire, Newhouse, and Sinaiko 2011). The act also extended the federal open enrollment period for Medigap plans to beneficiaries involuntarily disenrolling from MA plans under certain conditions such as the withdrawal of a plan from the market.

HEALTH INSURANCE AND THE USE OF MEDICAL CARE

This section discusses some basic principles in the economics of insurance design, and the next section will apply these concepts in the context of private insurance interacting with the Medicare program. While the main purpose of insurance is to protect consumers from financial risk associated with poor health, it can also affect patient incentives when seeking treatment. Getting sick or having an accident can be unpredictable, and the associated medical care is often very expensive. A person purchasing health insurance exchanges an upfront premium payment for compensation for medical care expenses if she gets sick in the future. People who are risk averse benefit from the reduction in uncertainty in their future financial resources.

When patients are fully reimbursed for their medical care spending, however, they and their physicians have little incentive to consider the cost of care when choosing among alternative treatments. In other words, by reducing the price of using medical care, insurance creates incentives for patients to use more care and more expensive care (Pauly 1968). Economists refer to this phenomenon as "moral hazard"—people behave differently when they have insurance than when they do not. The theoretical problem associated with moral hazard is not just that patients use more care, but that they use care that is costly relative to its benefits.

The Rand Health Insurance Experiment, a large randomized, controlled trial of the effects of health insurance on health care utilization and spending conducted in the 1970s, demonstrated that this effect is quantitatively important (Newhouse 1993). The study investigators randomly assigned people to health insurance plans with differing levels of cost sharing and then carefully tracked the quantity and type of medical care they used. People randomized to a 95 percent coinsurance plan—in other words, those who paid for nearly all their health care expenditures out of pocket—had 39 percent lower health care spending than those randomized to a "free care" plan that provided full coverage (Aron-Dine, Einav, and Finklestein 2013). While the Rand Health Insurance Experiment is considered the "gold standard" for estimating the effects of insurance coverage on the use of medical care owing to its rigorous study design, a large body of subsequent research using alternative methods reinforces the basic finding that more generous insurance coverage leads to greater utilization of medical care.

While moral hazard is simply the result of people responding to the financial incentives created by insurance, this type of behavior ultimately drives up health care spending. Because health insurance premiums reflect expected spending on covered services, increased utilization due to moral hazard is ultimately passed back to consumers in the form of higher premiums. In the case of private health insurance markets, higher premiums due to moral hazard make health insurance less affordable, resulting in fewer people purchasing coverage (Chernew, Cutler, and Keenan 2005). In the case of publicly financed care, the incremental cost is ultimately borne by taxpayers in the form of higher taxes or lower government spending on other types of services.

Because spending on low-value services ultimately makes coverage less attractive to consumers, private insurers have incentives to develop strategies to encourage patients and their providers to use care efficiently. One mechanism to control moral hazard in the use of insured health care is to require payments on the part of patients at the point of service. In other words, instead of fully reimbursing patients for the services they use, an insurer requires the patient to pay a portion of the amount billed by the provider at the point of service. The objective of this type of coinsurance or copayment is to reduce the use of low-value care by creating incentives for patients to consider the cost as well as the benefits of care when making treatment decisions.

Patient cost sharing, however, raises two types of concerns. First, it erodes the amount of protection that insurance provides. In other words, for consumers who initially purchased health insurance to protect themselves from financial risk, cost sharing at the point of service reintroduces financial risk associated with the use of health care. The optimal level of cost sharing balances these opposing effects (Zeckhauser 1970); patients give up some risk protection in exchange for lower premiums, reflecting less moral hazard in utilization. The second concern is that patients may not effectively discriminate between low- and high-value services when responding to cost sharing. Indeed, the Rand Health Insurance Experiment found that patients did not effectively discriminate between more and less appropriate care when reducing utilization (Newhouse 1993), and several studies have documented that patients with chronic conditions often discontinue the use of essential drugs in response to cost sharing, sometimes resulting in higher subsequent rates of hospitalization (Swartz 2010). In response, analysts have proposed differentiating the cost sharing for particular services based on the benefits relative to the costs. In particular, services for which the benefits are high relative to the costs would have low- or no-cost sharing (Fendrick et al. 2001).

Another mechanism that insurers use to influence utilization patterns is the structure of their relationships with providers. This type of mechanism, which is often referred to as managed care, includes a range of activities that are intended to influence how physicians, hospitals, and other types of providers deliver care. For example, hospitals and physicians can be paid in many different ways, ranging from a fee for each service they provide to a capitated payment for each patient under their care for a given time period. Fee-for-service payment, when the fee exceeds the marginal cost of care, creates incentives for hospitals and physicians to provide many services. Under capitation, in contrast, providers have incentives to do less. While these examples represent two extremes, more generally, insurers can influence provider behavior by designing payment systems that reward them financially for certain types of activities and penalize them for others. Insurers may also use nonfinancial mechanisms, such as giving physicians feedback on the utilization patterns of their patients relative to those of their peers or monitoring how their treatment patterns compare to clinical guidelines. Insurers adopting managed care mechanisms also usually contract with a subset of providers in a particular market.

Although the goal of managed care is to provide higher-quality and lower-cost care by discouraging the use of low-value services, similar to cost sharing, managed care mechanisms can pose some risks for consumers. The incentives that plans use to reduce the use of low-value care may also reduce the use of high-value care or create incentives for plans to avoid high-cost patients. In addition, while greater standardization of care processes may reduce the use of low-value services, it may also limit the extent to which plans accommodate differences across enrollees in either their clinical characteristics or their preferences for care.

Most private insurance plans use a combination of managed care and patient cost sharing to control moral hazard. When Medicare was enacted in 1965, the benefit resembled that of typical private health insurance at the time, relying primarily on patient cost sharing to control utilization, and the basic design of the coverage has changed relatively little since the program was established. The commercial market, in contrast, has changed dramatically since 1965, moving toward less patient cost sharing, more restricted provider networks, and greater use of managed care techniques. In 2011, the vast majority of the under-65 population was enrolled in a plan adopting restricted provider networks and incorporating at least some techniques of managed care (Claxton et al. 2011).

THE EFFECTS OF PRIVATE PLANS ON MEDICARE SPENDING

As the programs are currently designed, both types of private insurance have increased Medicare spending and thus have contributed to—

rather than alleviated—Medicare's spending issues. The mechanism by which they increase spending, however, differs.

Medigap

Medigap increases Medicare spending by covering the cost sharing of the traditional Medicare benefit. Insurers must offer coverage that conforms to 10 prespecified plans, and each plan is required to cover the Part A coinsurance as well as expenditures that exceed the benefit cap; most plans cover the Part B coinsurance and copayments (Table 7.1). The most popular plans, C and F, also cover the Part A and Part B deductibles. Thus, people with Medigap face little to no out-of-pocket payments for their Medicare-covered services.

While this benefit structure addresses an important weakness in the design of the traditional benefit, the coverage ceiling for inpatient care that exposes beneficiaries to significant financial risk, it also insulates beneficiaries from the financial consequence of their treatment decisions. For example, without Medigap insurance, a beneficiary would pay 20 percent of the price set by Medicare for a physician's office visit. With Medigap, however, the beneficiary is not required to make any out-of-pocket payment. The reduction in price, in theory, causes beneficiaries to use more care, although the magnitude of the effect depends on how responsive patients are to prices.

An important difference between primary and supplemental insurance is who bears the cost of the incremental utilization. When beneficiaries respond to lower out-of-pocket prices by using more care, the majority of the incremental expenditure is financed by the Medicare program, not the private insurer. Consider the example of the office visit discussed above. The private insurer covered only 20 percent of the price of the visit, while the Medicare program financed 80 percent. Thus, the premium charged by the private insurer reflects only a portion of the incremental expenditures generated by supplemental insurance, making Medigap look cheap to beneficiaries relative to the value of the services they receive. Private insurers usually prohibit enrollees from obtaining supplemental insurance for this reason.

While a number of studies have examined how supplemental insurance affects Medicare expenditures, the estimates of the magnitude of the effect vary from none to a 37 percent increase in Part B spending.

The range of estimates is perhaps not surprising, however, since the studies vary in many ways, encompassing different time periods with different regulatory environments and varying in the degree to which they distinguish Medigap from employer-sponsored retiree coverage and whether they adequately control for differences in health status between those who do and do not obtain coverage (Atherly 2001). Taken as a whole, however, the literature suggests that Medigap likely increases Medicare spending by approximately 15–25 percent.

In summary, while Medigap insurance provides beneficiaries with important financial protection, particularly given that beneficiaries are exposed to the possibility of very high out-of-pocket spending owing to a benefit cap for Part A services, it also counteracts the incentives for cost control in the design of the Medicare benefit. The incremental spending caused by supplemental insurance is financed in large part by the Medicare program.

Medicare Advantage

Although Medicare Part C was established to lower Medicare spending, the program instead has historically increased it, mainly because of the difficulty of setting payments for private plans in ways that both encourage enrollment and generate savings for Medicare (McGuire, Newhouse, and Sinaiko 2011). In the program's early years, the key issue was whether Medicare adequately adjusted the payments to private plans to reflect the health status of those choosing to enroll. When the program was established, the CMS set the payment to private plans at 95 percent of the average of Medicare spending for beneficiaries enrolled in traditional Medicare. Enrollment in an MA plan is voluntary, however, and those choosing to enroll have been, on average, in better health and thus less costly to insure than those choosing to remain in the traditional program. Initially, the CMS adjusted payments to plans using only a limited set of demographic characteristics, including age, sex, whether the beneficiary was also enrolled in Medicaid, whether the beneficiary was institutionalized, and whether the beneficiary was employed with employer-sponsored insurance (Pope et al. 2004). These characteristics, however, explained only a small portion of variation across beneficiaries in the annual expenditures—about 1 percent—raising the concern that the payments the CMS made for these enrollees exceeded what the cost would have been had the enrollees remained in the traditional program (Newhouse et al. 1989). Brown et al. (1993) find that it was indeed having that effect. Despite evidence that managed care plans reduced health care spending, particularly for less healthy enrollees, Medicare costs in the 1990s were 5.7 percent higher than they would have been in the absence of the MA program, owing to favorable selection.

In response to these concerns, the Balanced Budget Act of 1997 mandated that the CMS use a risk-adjustment methodology that incorporated enrollee health status when setting plan payments. In 2000, the CMS began risk adjusting payments using information on inpatient diagnoses (MedPAC 2005; Weissman, Wachterman, and Blumenthal 2005). Subsequent legislation mandated that by 2004 the CMS base its risk adjustment on data from both inpatient and ambulatory settings. This payment methodology was introduced gradually, with risk-adjusted payments representing 30, 50, and 75 percent of a blended rate in 2004, 2005, and 2006, respectively, and payments to plans were based entirely on a risk-adjusted rate beginning in 2007. While studies of the effect of the risk-adjustment methodology largely agree that the introduction of the payment methodology was associated with greater enrollment of less-healthy beneficiaries into MA plans (Brown et al. 2012; McWilliams, Hsu, and Newhouse 2012; Morrisey et al. 2012; Newhouse et al. 2012), the ultimate effect on Medicare spending is less clear. One study suggests that the more refined risk-adjustment system created greater scope for profitable favorable selection relative to payments. MA plans ultimately enrolled beneficiaries who were low cost relative to the payment formula with the result that overpayments to MA plans actually increased (Brown et al. 2012). Other research, however, has found that this dynamic had dissipated by 2008 (Newhouse et al. 2012).

In the later years of the program, the level of the average payment to MA plans, rather than the extent to which adjustments to the payment adequately compensated plans for difference in enrollee health status, became the primary focus of concerns over whether the MA program was increasing Medicare spending. In addition to requiring more detailed risk adjustment, the Balanced Budget Act of 1997 changed the payment formula to address differences between urban and rural areas, which had led to low rates of plan participation in rural areas.

The act set payment floors that essentially delinked county-level payments from historical spending levels. To offset the increase in Medicare expenditures due to the payment floors, which primarily affected rural counties, the legislation limited the rate of increase in payments in nonfloor counties. However, the payment floor had little effect on encouraging plans to enter rural counties, and the payment ceiling led plans in affected counties to reduce the generosity of the benefits they offered enrollees. As a result, the number of plans participating in MA and the number of beneficiaries enrolled declined dramatically between 1998 and 2002 (Figure 7.1).

Aiming to enhance the role of the private sector in Medicare, the Medicare Modernization Act of 2003 reversed this trend by increasing the average plan payment. The act stipulated that Medicare would pay the highest of an urban or rural floor payment, 100 percent of risk-adjusted per capita spending in Medicare, a minimum update over the prior year of 2 percent or traditional Medicare's national expenditure growth rate, and a blended payment (McGuire, Newhouse, and Sinaiko 2011). This formula guaranteed that average payment rates were at least as high as traditional Medicare spending in a particular county and locked in higher payments, even for counties experiencing relatively low-cost growth in the traditional Medicare program by linking the payment update to growth in national spending. MedPAC (2006) estimated that 2004 payments to MA plans averaged 107 percent of expected Medicare fee-for-service costs, not accounting for potential favorable selection. In 2006, Medicare instituted a system of plan bidding in which the CMS sets county-level benchmark payments and plans submit bids in response to the benchmarks. For plans submitting bids exceeding the benchmark, beneficiaries are responsible for paying the difference between the bid and the benchmark when enrolling. Plans bidding under the benchmark receive 75 percent of the difference as a rebate but must return the rebate to the beneficiaries in the form of additional benefits. Even after the implementation of the bidding system, MedPAC estimated that payments to MA were 111 percent of traditional Medicare costs (MedPAC 2006).

Figure 7.1 shows trends in plan participation and beneficiary enrollment in MA plans over time. Both enrollment and plan participation increased until the late 1990s, when plans began to exit the program in response to the rate reductions generated by the Balanced Budget Act of

Figure 7.1 Plan Participation and Beneficiary Enrollment in Medicare Advantage

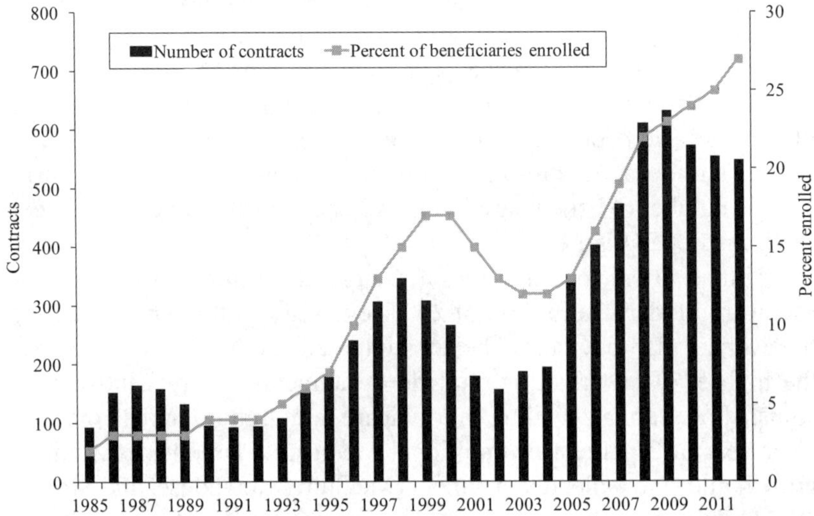

1997 and enrollment declined correspondingly. The payment increases generated by the Medicare Modernization Act of 2003 reversed the trend, with plan participation slowly increasing in early 2000 and then growing rapidly through 2009. Enrollment in MA plans increased correspondingly.

The history of the relationship between MA payment rates and plan participation and enrollment in MA plans demonstrates the tension policymakers face when trying to use the program both to provide beneficiaries with more choices and to control Medicare spending. When payments in urban areas rose less quickly during the late 1990s in order to contain program expenditures, plans dropped out of the program, the generosity of the benefits they offered declined, and enrollment declined correspondingly (Figure 7.1). When plan payments increased in the mid-2000s, plan participation and enrollment in the program increased, but so did Medicare spending. According to McGuire, Newhouse, and Sinaiko (2011), satisfying both these goals would require Medicare payment policy to "thread the policy needle."

THE FUTURE OF PRIVATE PLANS IN MEDICARE

What role should private plans play in Medicare's future? To date, Medigap and MA have exacerbated rather than alleviated Medicare's financing challenges by raising program costs. Yet, the more fundamental challenge is not simply to lower the rate of growth of program spending, but to provide Medicare-financed services more efficiently—to spend less but maintain or even improve quality of care. Achieving this objective, however, will require a significant change in how Medicare interacts with both providers and beneficiaries at the point of service. In the private insurance market, these relationships have evolved dramatically over time with the implementation of more sophisticated systems of patient cost sharing and the development of alternative ways of contracting with providers. The Medicare program, in contrast, has remained a relatively passive purchaser, paying providers mostly on a fee-for-service basis and providing few incentives for beneficiaries to consider both quality and cost when seeking care.

The Medicare program could achieve this transition through two types of approaches. First, it could reinvent itself as a more proactive purchaser of health care. In this scenario, the program would essentially be reformed from the inside by redesigning provider payment methods to promote the delivery of high-value care and restructuring the benefit package to engage patients more fully in considering both cost and quality of treatment decisions. The program has already taken steps in this direction in recent years, particularly in its relationships with providers, through the development of quality reporting systems and pay-for-performance for particular types of services (Tanenbaum 2009). The ACA contains a number of provisions that continue this approach (James 2012). Perhaps the most well-known example is the establishment of Accountable Care Organizations (ACOs), which are groups of providers that agree to be held responsible for a defined group of beneficiaries and are rewarded financially if the Medicare expenditures for the group are lower than projected. The act also introduced a program designed to reduce potentially avoidable hospital readmissions. Under the current fee-for-service system, hospitals have little financial incentive to invest in after-discharge follow-up care, which would prevent future admissions, since they do not benefit financially from these activities, and even potentially forego the profit associated with the future admission. Hospitals are now financially penalized for high readmission rates (Joynt and Jha 2013).

Medicare is the largest purchaser of health services in the country, and its size makes this approach more feasible, since the program has the purchasing leverage to drive substantive change in provider practice. For example, after Medicare adopted prospective payment for inpatient hospital admission in the 1980s, many private insurers soon followed, negotiating prices based on the diagnosis-related group definitions used by the CMS. While Medicare's sheer size may be an advantage in creating incentives for providers to adopt new payment methods or other types of innovations, such as electronic medical records, its role as a governmental organization creates other types of barriers. While some express concern over whether a government-run monopoly can be adequately incentivized to produce services efficiently, another important difference between public and private insurers is the political pressure they face. In addition to the enrollees who rely on the program for their health care, Medicare is beholden to a variety of stakeholders because of the size of the program relative to the overall economy. Medicare administrative decisions can have dramatic financial consequences for physicians, hospitals, pharmaceutical companies, device manufacturers, local governments, and others, leading to continuous congressional involvement in the program as representatives respond to their particular set of constituents. Kessler (2012) proposes that Medicare's vulnerability to congressional micromanagement makes the program fundamentally unable to make the difficult decisions that would be required to relentlessly focus on the delivery of high-value care. Perhaps the most visible example of how politics affects the operation of the program is the development of physician reimbursement policy. As part of the Balanced Budget Act of 1997, Congress reformed physician payment policy by linking fee increases to an expenditure target in order to contain physician expenditures (Congressional Budget Office 2006). However, every year since 2003, Congress has blocked the formula from taking effect, since it would substantially reduce physician fees, potentially threatening beneficiaries' access to care (Jacobs 2013). Although many policymakers agree that the formula needs to be fixed to create a more stable, long-term payment policy, there has not yet been bipartisan agreement on a solution.

The primary alternative to "reform from within" is to restructure Medicare as a marketplace of government-subsidized, regulated private plans, a model often referred to as "premium support." Rather than receive an open-ended guarantee to cover all medically necessary services, beneficiaries would instead receive a fixed payment in the form of a voucher for a defined set of services and could direct the payment to the private plan of their choice (MedPAC 2013a). While this approach is attractive from a government budgeting perspective because it provides policymakers with more control over Medicare spending through control of the voucher size, its theoretical rationale is based on the potential benefits of competition among health plans as a mechanism to promote efficient utilization of care. A voucher would expose beneficiaries to the higher costs of more expensive plans, introducing price sensitivity at the point of insurance purchase. Competition among plans for enrollees, in turn, would create incentives for plans to develop mechanisms to control cost and increase quality of care. This is an important deviation from the existing Medicare program because it rewards beneficiaries for using care more parsimoniously through their choice of a lower-premium plan. This approach also creates the opportunity for variation across plans in both the generosity of benefits and the structure of delivery system, allowing for better customization of care for individual preferences. From a political economy perspective, premium support shifts the responsibility for implementing managed care mechanisms from the public to the private sector, creating less opportunity for political interference in plan management (Kessler 2012).

Opponents of premium support raise two types of concerns. First, while the intent is to harness the power of competition to provide more effective care, plans may compete in less socially beneficial ways, such as by trying to enroll beneficiaries in better health or by withholding access to beneficial care. While the policy response to the potential for risk selection is to adjust payments to plans to reflect differences among enrollees in their expected costs, whether existing systems of risk adjustment adequately ameliorate these incentives remains an open question (Brown et al. 2012; McWilliams, Hsu, and Newhouse 2012). In the case of concerns over "stinting," the policy response is to provide consumers with information on plan quality. This would provide a mechanism for the market to reward high-quality plans in the form of higher rates of enrollment. As in the case of risk adjustment, although the availability of this type of information has increased dramatically in recent years, there is still some uncertainty over whether this approach would adequately address these types of concerns.

The other concern from the perspective of beneficiaries is the extent to which premium support shifts responsibility for financing health care from taxpayers to beneficiaries. This depends primarily on how the level of the voucher is set. The amount the government contributes could be chosen administratively, as it has been traditionally done in the MA program, or it could be determined through a market process (MedPAC 2013b). If the level of the voucher is set administratively, then a key issue is how the voucher is adjusted over time. Because increases in health care costs typically exceed inflation, linking the level of the voucher to the rate of growth of the economy as a whole would transfer an increasing portion of financing of health care costs to beneficiaries over time. Voucher amounts linked to growth in health care spending, in contrast, provide greater protection for beneficiaries against health care cost growth. An alternative is to set the level of the voucher through a competitive process. In Medicare Part D, plans submit bids for covering beneficiaries, and the subsidy is calculated as a share of the average national bid. Linking the subsidy to a market-determined level of health care spending protects beneficiaries from market trends specific to health care.

Medicare beneficiaries have had a private alternative to the traditional benefit for nearly 20 years, however, so why has Medicare Part C not been more successful in generating greater value from Medicare-financed services? The current program suffers not necessarily from the inability of private plans to provide care more efficiently but from the lack of incentives for beneficiaries to seek out more efficient alternatives. One reason is that MA plans are limited in the ways in which they are able to transfer any savings they generate to beneficiaries. In particular, they may not pay beneficiaries to enroll. Instead, they must transfer any cost savings they generate to beneficiaries in the form of additional benefits. This results in the provision of products and services of relatively low value to beneficiaries and lessens plans' incentives to provide care more efficiently. Another reason is that MA plans currently compete not against just traditional Medicare but against the combination of Medicare and supplemental insurance. As discussed earlier, however, much of the incremental utilization associated with supplemental insurance is financed by the Medicare program, making premiums for supplemental coverage low relative to the benefits it provides. The relative attractiveness to beneficiaries of traditional Medicare plus Medigap, which is financed primarily by taxpayers, makes MA plans less attractive.

Not only does the availability of Medigap coverage limit enrollment in MA plans, but it also weakens the likely effectiveness of "reform from within" by essentially taking patient cost sharing off the table as a mechanism to influence utilization of care. For example, the financial incentives of ACOs, while intended to create incentives for these organizations to provide care more efficiently, also create a tension between beneficiaries and providers. The savings associated with lower utilization of care ultimately benefit providers and taxpayers rather than beneficiaries themselves, since they have little to no cost sharing and thus do not experience a decline in their out-of-pocket spending. Helchem et al. (2013) propose a "shared-savings supplement" in which beneficiaries would receive a cash payment for choosing a lower cost option to restore patient incentives in the face of supplemental insurance.

The implication of the interrelationships between Medigap and the traditional program is that effective reform of the Medicare program will also require reform of the Medigap market. The tension in reforming this market, however, is how to provide beneficiaries with catastrophic risk protection while limiting the extent to which that protection promotes inefficient use of care. One potential approach is to restructure the cost sharing associated with traditional Medicare. For example, MedPAC has recommended redesigning the traditional Medicare benefit by creating an out-of-pocket maximum for cost sharing, maintaining the Part A and B deductibles (and possibly combining them into a single deductible), replacing coinsurance with copayments for most services, and allowing the secretary to adjust the cost sharing for specific services based on their value to patients (MedPAC 2012b). With this type of restructuring, the basic benefit would provide beneficiaries protection from large expenditures but retain incentives for them to avoid low-value care.

While improving the benefit design of the traditional Medicare program would likely reduce demand for supplemental coverage, reform of the Medigap market may be necessary as well. In general, Medigap reform should be guided by the objective of limiting the extent to which the incremental costs associated with the purchase of supplemental insurance are borne by taxpayers rather than beneficiaries. In particular, policymakers could restrict Medigap plans from providing first-dollar coverage or require them to apply copayments for certain services. Alternatively, they could tax plans providing first-dollar coverage or charge Medicare beneficiaries a fee if they purchase supplemental insurance, where the tax or the fee reflected the incremental cost the coverage generates for the Medicare program.

CONCLUSION

To date, private health insurance has done little to improve the efficiency of the delivery of Medicare-financed services and has actually increased Medicare spending. Medigap insurance has aggravated the inefficiencies associated with traditional Medicare coverage, and while MA plans have the potential to improve the efficiency of service delivery, the design of the Part C benefit limits the ability of plans to pass these efficiencies on to enrollees, and the availability of Medigap coverage further dilutes the incentives of beneficiaries to enroll in plans that provide care more efficiently. While private plans have the potential to be part of solutions to Medicare's budget challenges, this would require reform to the traditional Medicare program, the supplemental insurance market, and the MA program.

References

Aron-Dine, Aviva, Liran Einav, and Amy Finklestein. 2013. "The RAND Health Insurance Experiment, Three Decades Later." *Journal of Economic Perspectives* 27(1): 197–222.

Atherly, Adam. 2001. "Supplemental Insurance: Medicare's Accidental Stepchild." *Medical Care Research and Review* 58(2): 131–161.

Baicker, Katherine, and Amitabh Chandra. 2004. "Medicare Spending, the Physician Workforce, and Beneficiaries' Quality of Care." *Health Affairs* Web Exclusives: W4-184–197. doi:10.1377/hlthaff.w4.184 (accessed September 2, 2015).

Brown, Jason, Mark Duggan, Ilyana Kuziemko, and William Woolston. 2012. "How Does Risk Selection Respond to Risk Adjustment? New Evidence from the Medicare Advantage Program." Columbia Business School Working Paper. New York: Columbia University. https://www0.gsb.columbia.edu/faculty/ikuziemko/papers/ma_draft_18oct2012_ik.pdf (accessed September 2, 2015).

Brown, Randall S., Dolores Gurnick Clement, Jerrold W. Hill, Sheldon M. Retchin, and Jeanette W. Bergeron. 1993. "Do Health Maintenance Organizations Work for Medicare?" *Health Care Financing Review* 15(1): 7–23.

Cafferata, Gail Lee. 1985. "Private Health Insurance of the Medicare Population and the Baucus Legislation." *Medical Care* 23(9): 1086–1096.

Chandra, Amitabh, Jonathan Holmes, and Jonathan Skinner. 2013. "Is This Time Different? The Slowdown in Healthcare Spending." Brookings Papers on Economic Activity. Washington, DC: Brookings Institution.

Chernew, Michael, David M. Cutler, and Patricia Seliger Keenan. 2005. "Increasing Health Insurance Costs and the Decline in Health Insurance Coverage." *Health Services Research* 40(4): 1021–1039.

Claxton, Gary, Matthew Rae, Nirmita Panchal, Janet Lundy, Anthony Damico, Awo Osei-Anto, Kevin Kenward, Heidi Whitmore, and Jeremy Pickreign. 2011. "Employer Health Benefits: 2011 Annual Survey." Menlo Park, CA: Henry J. Kaiser Foundation and Chicago: Health Research & Educational Trust.

Congressional Budget Office. 2006. "The Sustainable Growth Rate Formula for Setting Medicare's Physician Payment Rates." Economic and Budget Issue Brief, September 6. Washington, DC: CBO. https://www.cbo.gov/sites/default/files/109th-congress-2005-2006/reports/09-07-sgr-brief.pdf (accessed September 2, 2015).

———. 2013. Updated Budget Projections: Fiscal Years 2013 to 2023. Washington, DC: CBO. https://www.cbo.gov/sites/default/files/cbofiles/attachments/44172-Baseline2.pdf (accessed September 2, 2015).

Cutler, David M. 2004. *Your Money or Your Life: Strong Medicine for America's Health Care System*. New York: Oxford University Press.

Fendrick, A. Mark, Dean G. Smith, Michael E. Chernew, and Sonali N. Shah. 2001. "A Benefit-Based Copay for Prescription Drugs: Patient Contribution Based on Total Benefits, Not Drug Acquisition Cost." *American Journal of Managed Care* 7(9): 861–867.

Fisher, Elliott S., David E. Wennberg, Thrse A. Stukel, Daniel J. Gottlieb, F. L. Lucas, and Étoile L. Pinder. 2003. "The Implications of Regional Variations in Medicare Spending." Parts 1 and 2. *Annals of Internal Medicine* 138(4): 273–298.

Fox, Peter D., Thomas Rice, and Lisa Alecxih. 1995. "Medigap Regulation: Lessons for Health Care Reform." *Journal of Health Politics, Policy and Law* 20(1): 31–48.

Fuchs, Victor R. 1996. "Economic Values and Healthcare Reform." *American Economic Review* 86(1): 125–148.

Government Accountability Office. 1986. "Medigap Insurance: Law Has Increased Protection against Substandard and Overpriced Policies." Washington, DC: USGAO. http://www.gao.gov/assets/150/144800.pdf (accessed September 2, 2015).

Hall, Robert E., and Charles I. Jones. 2007. "The Value of Life and the Rise in Health Spending." *Quarterly Journal of Economics* 122(1): 39–72.

Helchem, Lorens A., William E. Encinosa, Michael E. Chernew, and Richard A. Hirth. 2013. "Integrating Patient Incentives with Episode-Based Payment." *Forum for Health Economics and Policy* 16(1): 1–14.

Institute of Medicine. 2011. "The Healthcare Imperative: Lowering Costs and Improving Outcomes: Workshop Series Summary." Learning Health System Series. Washington, DC: National Research Council.

———. 2013. *Interim Report of the Committee on Geographic Variation in Health Care Spending and Promotion of High-Value Health Care: Preliminary Committee Observations.* Washington, DC: National Research Council.

Jacobs, Chris. 2013. "Medicare's Sustainable Growth Rate: Principles for Reform." Backgrounder No. 2827. Washington, DC: Heritage Foundation. http://www.heritage.org/research/reports/2013/07/medicares-sustainable-growth-rate-principles-for-reform (accessed September 2, 2015).

James, Julia. 2012. "Pay-for-Performance. New Payment Systems Reward Doctors and Hospitals for Improving the Quality of Care, but Studies to Date Show Mixed Results." Health Policy Brief. *Health Affairs*, October 11.

Joynt, Karen E., and Ashish K. Jha. 2013. "A Path Forward on Medicare Readmissions." *New England Journal of Medicine* 368(13): 1175–1177.

Kaiser Family Foundation. 2011. Kaiser Health Tracking Poll: Public Opinion on Health Care Issues. Menlo Park, CA: Henry J. Kaiser Family Foundation. https://kaiserfamilyfoundation.files.wordpress.com/2013/01/8217-f.pdf (accessed September 2, 2015).

———. 2012. "Medicare at a Glance." Menlo Park, CA: Henry J. Kaiser Family Foundation. http://kff.org/medicare/fact-sheet/medicare-at-a-glance-fact-sheet (accessed November 19, 2013).

Kessler, Daniel P. 2012. "Real Medicare Reform." *National Review* 13(Fall 2012). http://www.nationalaffairs.com/publications/detail/real-medicare-reform (accessed September 2, 2015).

Lew, Jacob J., Kathleen Sebelius, Charles P. Blahous III, Seth D. Harris, Carolyn W. Colvin, Robert D. Reischauer, and Marilyn B. Tavenner. 2013. *2013 Annual Report of the Boards of Trustees of the Federal Hospital Insurance and Federal Supplementary Medical Insurance Trust Funds.* Washington, DC: Boards of Trustees, Federal Hospital Insurance and Federal Supplementary Medical Insurance Trust Funds.

McCall, Nelda, Thomas Rice, and Arden Hall. 1987. "The Effect of State Regulations on the Quality and Sale of Insurance Policies to Medicare Beneficiaries." *Journal of Health Politics, Policy and Law* 12(1): 53–76.

McCall, Nelda, Thomas Rice, and Judith Sangl. 1986. "Consumer Knowledge of Medicare and Supplemental Health Insurance Benefits." *Health Services Research* 20(6): 633–657.

McCormack, Lauren A., Peter D. Fox, Thomas Rice, and Marcia L. Graham. 1996. "Medigap Reform Legislation of 1990: Have the Objectives Been Met?" *Health Care Financing Review* 18(1): 157–173.

McGuire, Thomas G., Joseph P. Newhouse, and Anna D. Sinaiko. 2011. "An Economic History of Medicare Part C." *Milbank Quarterly* 89(2): 289–332.

McWilliams, J. Michael, John Hsu, and Joseph P. Newhouse. 2012. "New Risk-Adjustment System Was Associated with Reduced Favorable Selection in Medicare Advantage." *Health Affairs* 31(12): 2630–2640.

Medicare Payment Advisory Commission (MedPAC). 2005. "Issues in a Modernized Medicare Program." Report to Congress. Washington, DC: MedPAC. http://www.medpac.gov/documents/reports/June05_Entire_report.pdf?sfvrsn=0 (accessed September 2, 2015).

———. 2006. "Medicare Advantage Benchmarks and Payments Compared with Average Medicare Fee-for-Service Spending." *Medicare Briefs*. Washington, DC: MedPAC. http://www.pnhp.org/single_payer_resources/medicare_overpayments.pdf (accessed September 2, 2015).

———. 2011. "Medicare and the Health Care Delivery System." Report to Congress. Washington, DC: MedPAC. http://www.medpac.gov/documents/reports/Jun11_EntireReport.pdf?sfvrsn=0 (accessed September 2, 2015).

———. 2013a. "Part D Payment System." *Payment Basics*. Washington, DC: MedPAC.

———. 2013b. "Medicare and the Health Care Delivery System." Report to Congress. Washington, DC: MedPAC. http://medpac.gov/documents/reports/jun13_entirereport.pdf?sfvrsn=0 (accessed September 2, 2015).

Moon, Marilyn. 1996. "What Medicare Has Meant to Older Americans." *Health Care Financing Review* 18(2): 49–59.

Morrisey, Michael A., Meredith L. Kilgore, David J. Becker, Wilson Smith, and Elizabeth Delzell. 2012. "Favorable Selection, Risk Adjustment, and the Medicare Advantage Program." *Health Services Research* 48(3): 1039–1056.

Newhouse, Joseph P. 1993. *Free for All? Lessons from the RAND Health Insurance Experiment.* Cambridge, MA: Harvard University Press.

Newhouse, Joseph P., Willard G. Manning, Emmett B. Keeler, and Elizabeth M. Sloss. 1989. "Adjusting Capitation Rates Using Objective Health Measures and Prior Utilization." *Health Care Financing Review* 10(3): 41–53.

Newhouse, Joseph P., Mary Price, Jie Huang, J. Michael Williams, and John Hsu. 2012. "Steps to Reduce Favorable Risk Selection in Medicare Advantage Largely Succeeded, Boding Well for Health Insurance Exchanges." *Health Affairs* 31(12): 2618–2628.

Pauly, M. V. 1968. "The Economics of Moral Hazard: Comment (with Further Comment by K. J. Arrow)." *American Economic Review* 58(3): 531–539.

Pope, Gregory C., John Kautter, Randall P. Ellis, Arlene S. Ash, John Z. Ayanian, Lisa I. Iezzoni, Melvin J. Ingber, Jesse M. Levy, and John Robst. 2004. "Risk Adjustment of Medicare Capitation Payments Using the CMS-HCC Model." *Health Care Financing Review* 25(4): 119–141.

Remler, Dahlia K., and Sherry A. Glied. 2003. "What Other Programs Can Teach Us: Increasing Participation in Health Insurance Programs." *American Journal of Public Health* 93(1): 67–74.

Skinner, Jonathan S., Douglas O. Staiger, and Elliott S. Fisher. 2006. "Is Technological Change in Medicine Always Worth It? The Case of Acute Myocardial Infarction." *Health Affairs* 25(2): w34–w47.

Swartz, Katherine. 2010. *Cost-Sharing: Effects on Spending and Outcomes.* Research Synthesis Report No. 20. Princeton, NJ: The Synthesis Project, Robert Wood Johnson Foundation. http://www.rwjf.org/content/dam/farm/reports/issue_briefs/2010/rwjf402103/subassets/rwjf402103_1 (accessed September 3, 2015).

Tanenbaum, Sandra J. 2009. "Pay for Performance in Medicare: Evidentiary Irony and the Politics of Value." *Journal of Health Politics, Policy and Law* 34(5): 717–746.

Weissman, Joel S., Melissa Wachterman, and David Blumenthal. 2005. "When Methods Meet Politics: How Risk Adjustment Became Part of Medicare Managed Care." *Journal of Health Politics, Policy and Law* 30(3): 475–504.

Zeckhauser, Richard. 1970. "Medical Insurance: A Case Study of the Tradeoff between Risk Spreading and Appropriate Incentives." *Journal of Economic Theory* 2(1): 10–26.

Authors

M. Kate Bundorf is an associate professor at Stanford University.

Marcus Dillender is an economist at the W.E. Upjohn Institute for Employment Research.

John H. Goddeeris is a professor at Michigan State University.

Donald J. Meyer is chair of the Department of Economics and a professor at Western Michigan University.

Edward C. Norton is a professor at the University of Michigan and a research associate at the National Bureau of Economic Research.

Charles E. Phelps is a professor and provost emeritus at the University of Rochester.

Index

Note: The italic letters *f*, *n*, or *t* following a page number indicate a figure, note, or table, respectively, on that page. Double letters mean more than one such item on a single page.

ACA. *See* Patient Protection and Affordable Care Act
Accidents, 15, 15*f*, 35
Accountable care organizations (ACOs), 4, 54–55, 61–70
- comprehensive care responsibility proposed for, 4, 61–64
- language of, included in ACA, 61, 74*n*4
- managed competition and, 65–70, 71, 76*n*13
- Medicare payment reform through, 54–55, 71, 137
- regulation or competition by, 64–65

Addiction prevention, 24–25
Adverse selection, 114
- mitigation of, 110, 111
- moral hazard and, 2, 5, 105
- problem of, on health insurance purchases, 103, 110

African countries, complementary health care in developing, 45–46
Aging. *See* Population pyramids
Alcohol consumption, 25, 48
- as actual cause of death, 3, 15*f*, 22
- distilled spirits *vs.* wine, 20, 28, 31*nn*5–6
- levels of education and, 28–29, 30*f*

Alternative Quality Contract (AQC)
- consumer choice and, 69–70
- quality care and, 64–65, 74*n*6, 133, 137

Australia, medical spending in, 7, 8*f*, 9*f*, 10*f*
Austria, medical spending in, 8*f*, 9*f*, 10*f*

Balanced Budget Act, 124, 130, 131, 134
BCBS. *See* Blue Cross Blue Shield
Belgium, medical spending in, 8*f*, 9*f*, 10*f*
Bending the curve. *See* Health care spending, reduction of
Benefits
- cash and counseling, 106, 108, 110
- disability, 88*f*, 92–93
- eligibility for, 86–87, 92, 107, 108, 110, 120
- fringe, 1, 29, 43, 81, 92, 118, 129
- indemnity, 92–93, 93*f*
- medical, 5, 61, 93, 93*f*, 119–120
- prescription drugs, 5, 66, 69, 73, 76*n*13, 120
- Social Security, 113

Blue Cross Blue Shield (BCBS)
- of Massachusetts, 64–65, 69–70, 74*n*4
- of Michigan, 43–44

Body mass index (BMI)
- calculations of, 17–20, 31*nn*3–4
- lowering of, as change, 24, 28, 31*n*8, 48
- quality of life and, 20, 21*ff*

Bundled Payments for Care Improvement (BPCI), as Medicare mandate, 59–60

Canada, medical spending in, 7, 8*f*, 9*f*, 10*f*
Capitation
- as basis for health care payments, 60–61, 112, 126–127
- differences of, from ACO payments, 61–62
- Medicare Part C and, 66, 69, 122

CBO oversight. *See* Congressional Budget Office oversight
Centers for Medicaid and Medicare Services (CMS), functions of, 119, 122, 124, 129–130, 131, 134

China, educational attainment in, 26
Chronic diseases. *See* Diseases deemed chronic
Cigarette smoking, 22
  as actual cause of death, 16*f,* 20
  quality of life and, 20, 21*ff*
  reduction of, and culture change, 16–17, 16*f,* 23, 27–28, 27*f,* 30*n*2
CLASS Act. *See* Community Living Assistance Services and Supports Act
CMS. *See* Centers for Medicaid and Medicare Services
Cocaine, 20, 22
College graduates. *See* Educational levels; Postsecondary educational attainment
Community Living Assistance Services and Supports (CLASS) Act, 5, 103–114
  background issues of, 104–106
  economic problems of, 109–114
  purpose and provisions of, 103, 106–109
  summary of, 5, 114
Competition, 111
  cost control, for quality care, 69, 135
  economic, 26
  managed, and ACOs, 65–70, 75*n*6
  market-based, and health care spending, 55–56
  regulation or, and ACOs, 64–65
Congressional Budget Office (CBO) oversight
  CLASS Act and, 103, 108–109
  health care spending and, 52–53, 74*n*1, 83
Consumer choices, 71, 105, 127
  AQC and, 69–70
  CLASS Act and, 106, 107, 113
  health care decision making and, 55–56, 60, 65, 68, 74*n*3, 75*nn*10–11
  trade-offs in, 72, 73*f,* 74, 133
Czech Republic, medical spending in, 8*f,* 9*f,* 10*f*
Dartmouth College, health care spending research at, 54, 74*n*4
Death, 22, 24, 25
  leading causes of, among lifestyle choices, 3, 14–15, 15*f*
  spirals of, and asymmetric information, 2, 103
  See also Mortality rates
Denmark, 20
  medical spending in, 8*f,* 9*f,* 10*f*
Dental care, Medicare and, 118
Diet. *See* Food consumption and diet
Disability insurance, 119
  nature and purpose of, 4–5, 81, 86–88
  potential effects of ACA on, 81–82, 88–92, 96–98
  SSDI and SSI components of, 86–88, 88*f,* 89*f,* 90–91
  See also Workers' compensation insurance
Diseases deemed chronic
  cancers, 15, 16, 19, 20, 22, 25
  diabetes, 19, 44
  heart conditions, 19, 20, 23, 25, 44, 46
  hypertension, 19, 44
  stroke, 22, 23, 25
Drugs
  addictive, and national research institutes, 25
  See also Illicit drugs; Over-the-counter drugs; Prescription drugs

Economic factors
  asymmetric information in health markets as, 2–3, 110
  goods and services in health modeling, 1–2, 58–60
Education levels
  healthy lifestyle improvement by, 3, 26–30, 27*f,* 29*f,* 30*f,* 31*n*9
  influence of, on health, 2, 6
Elderly population, 96
  cash and counseling programs for needy, 106, 108
  health care spending and, 53, 117
  long-term care and, 5, 104–105, 110

Elderly population, *cont.*
in U.S. population pyramids, 10–11, 12*ff*–13*ff*
Employer responsibility, 113, 118
ACA mandate for, 1, 82, 84*t*
Employment fringe benefits, 1, 92
health insurance, 29, 43, 81, 118, 129
End-stage renal disease, Medicare coverage of, 119
Enthoven, Alain, managed competition and, 65
Environment, influence on health, 2
EPI. *See* Expanded Programme on Immunization
European paradox, lifestyle choices and, 22–23
Exercise activity, 3, 44, 48
Expanded Programme on Immunization (EPI), UN initiative, 45–46

FDA. *See* Food and Drug Administration
Fee-for-service, 61
capitation *vs.*, 60, 70–71, 126–127
health care spending as, 54, 56–58
mathematical equations for Medicare payments to ACOs, 62–64, 74–75*n*5
Finland, medical spending in, 8*f*, 9*f*, 10*f*
Fisher, Elliot, 54
ACOs and, 61, 74*n*4
Food and Drug Administration (FDA), drug approvals by, 24
Food consumption and diet
as actual cause of death, 15*f*, 18–19, 19*f*, 31*n*4
healthy eating, 23, 48
as poor lifestyle choice and death, 3, 9
France, medical spending in, 8*f*, 9*f*, 10*f*

GDP. *See* Gross domestic product
Gender differences, 20, 48
obesity rates and, 28, 29*f*
in population pyramids, 10–11, 12*ff*–13*ff*
Germany, medical spending in, 7, 8*f*, 9*f*, 10*f*
Ghana, substitution and complementarity care effects in, 47
Government roles, 134
address problems that private market cannot, 110–111
regulation, 24, 64–65, 121–122, 129
Greece, medical spending in, 8*f*, 9*f*, 10*f*
Gross domestic product (GDP), per capita, and health care spending, 7, 51–54, 52*f*

Hackbarth, Glenn, ACOs and, 74*n*4
Harvard University, fee-for-service study at, 56–57
Health
factors and types of care that influence, 2, 35–38
good, as output, 1, 60
improved, with health insurance, 97, 98
modeling, with economic factors, 1–2, 37, 58–60
relationship between, and health spending, 72–73, 73*f*, 76*n*14, 117
Health care, 30*n*1, 53
government systems for, 7, 29–30, 47
managed, and spending, 60, 67–68, 75*n*9, 126, 130
outcomes of delivered services for, 8–9, 118, 133
positive spillovers in, 47–48
types of, 2, 35–38
(*see also* Medical care; Self-care)
uncertainty and, 38–44, 104
Health care spending
on chronic diseases, 11, 14*f*, 19, 20, 22
compared to Social Security spending, 53, 53*f*
excess cost growth in, 53, 74*n*1
financial incentives in, 29, 43, 56–58, 65, 71, 124–126
GDP per capita and, 7, 11, 36, 54, 117
global, 1, 3, 6, 7–10, 8*f*, 9*f*, 10*f*
patient cost sharing in, 104, 105, 126–127, 128, 133

Health care spending, *cont.*
reduction of, 24, 48, 51–55, 52*f,* 70, 72–74, 73*f*
relationship between, and health, 72–73, 73*f,* 76*n*14, 117
waste prevention in, 72, 73*f,* 86
See also under Medical care, spending for; Medicare program, spending for
Health insurance, 55, 103
challenges in, 2–3, 5, 53–54
employer-paid, 29, 43, 81, 118, 129
improved health with, 97–98
mechanism of coverage by, 29, 42–44
risk pools in, 61, 75*n*7
role of private, in Medicare, 5, 118–119, 120–124, 127–136
self-financed, 103, 107
state exchanges for, 1, 43, 67, 70, 74, 75*n*8, 76*n*13, 81, 83
use of medical care in, 124–127
See also Medicare program; Private health insurance
Health maintenance organizations (HMOs)
Massachusetts BCBS among, 65, 69–70
payment for managed care by, 56, 60–61
Health markets
asymmetric information and, 2–3, 55–56, 110
bundling in, 59–60, 74*n*3, 75*n*6
comprehensive care in, 60–70 (*see also* Accountable care organizations (ACOs))
cost and quality trade-offs in, 72, 73*f,* 74
fee-for-service in, 56–58
payments to providers in, 54–60, 74*n*3, 75*n*6, 96, 126–127, 133
various ACA measures in, 83, 85*t,* 86
Heroin, 20, 22
HHS. *See* U.S. Dept. of Health and Human Services
High-income population, 72, 105, 117, 120
High school graduates. *See* Educational levels
HMOs. *See* Health maintenance organizations
Home health care, 104, 105–106, 112
Hospitalization, 35, 58, 108
admission incentives for, 86, 126, 133–134
public insurance for, payments, 5, 22, 59, 62
Hungary, medical spending in, 8*f,* 9*f,* 10*f*

Iceland, medical spending in, 8*f,* 9*f,* 10*f*
Illicit drugs, 15, 15*f,* 20, 22
Illness, 24, 35
Income
elasticity of, and health care, 30*n*1, 108
relationship between, and medical spending, 3, 7–8, 8*f*
See also High-income population; Low-income population
Indemnity benefits, 92–93, 93*f*
Independent Payment Advisory Board (IPAB), Medicare cost-cutting and, 83, 91, 96
India, educational attainment in, 26
Individual mandate. *See under* Personal responsibility, mandate for
Infant mortality, relationship between, and medical spending, 3, 9, 10*f,* 54
Inflation risk, long-term care insurance and, 5, 112
Injuries, 24, 35, 105
on-the-job, and workers compensation insurance, 4–5, 81, 92, 94, 95, 96
Insurance markets, 74*n*6, 112
challenges in all, 5, 39
contract functions in, 39–40, 122–124, 127
copayments and deductibles in, 104, 105, 126, 137

Insurance markets, *cont.*
creation of, for long-term care, 103, 106
government role in, when private entities cannot address problems, 110–111
Integrated practice units, 65, 74*n*6
Internal Revenue Service (IRS), payroll deduction policies of, 113
IPAB. *See* Independent Payment Advisory Board
Ireland, medical spending in, 8*f,* 9*f,* 10*f*
IRS. *See* Internal Revenue Service
Italy, medical spending in, 8*f,* 9*f,* 10*f*

Japan, 22
life expectancy and medical spending in, 8–9, 9*f*
other medical spending in, 7, 8*f,* 10*f*
Johnson, Pres. Lyndon, war on chronic diseases and, 25

K–12 educational attainment, 26, 27
U.S. alcohol use by, 28, 30*f*
U.S. obesity rates and, 28, 29*f*
U.S. smokers with, 27*f,* 28
Kaiser Permanente health plan, capitation for managed care in, 60

Labor force, 24, 113
See also Working-age population
Life expectancy
gender differences in, 11, 12*ff*–13*ff*
relationship between, and medical spending, 3, 8–9, 9*f,* 52, 54
Lifestyle choices, 3, 14–29
fixing poor choices, 3, 23–29
improvement of, through education, 26–30, 31*n*9
poor, and managing adverse health consequences, 24–26
self-care and, 2, 27, 44
Liver diseases, Medicare coverage of, 20
Long-term care
alternatives to formal, 105–106
dropped from ACA legislation, 5, 103–104
Medicare limited for, 104, 118
private market for, insurance, 109–110, 111, 112
voluntary insurance for, 103, 106–107, 111
Lou Gehrig's disease, Medicare coverage of, 119
Low-income population
cash and counseling programs for elderly, 106, 108
Medicaid and supplemental coverage for, 118, 120
SSI beneficiaries as, 86–87, 89*f*
subsets of, exempted from ACA mandate, 83, 85*t*
subsidies for, purchase of health insurance, 81, 83

Malawi, EPI and maternal care complementarity in, 45–46
Marijuana, 20, 22
Massachusetts, health insurance in, 64–65, 69–70, 74*n*4, 94
Medicaid program, 20, 111, 118
expansion of, in ACA, 1, 43, 81, 83, 85*t,* 108
help with copayments and deductibles in, 104, 105, 137
Medical care
services for, and health, 2, 58, 97, 98
sole use of, or in combination with self-care, 3–4, 35–36, 42–44, 46–48
spending for, 3, 5, 22, 93, 93*f*
as substitute, with poor choices, 45, 46
use of, in health insurance, 124–127
Medicare Advantage plans, 69
CMS and, 122, 124, 130–131
Medicare spending and enrollment, 129–132, 132*f*
premium support in, 136–137
as private replacement Part C in Medicare, 5, 66–67, 75*n*7, 120, 122, 124

Medicare Advantage plans, *cont.*
risk adjustment and, 68, 71, 76*n*12, 124
Medicare Modernization Act
payment plans changed by, and Part C, 131–132, 132*f*
Prescription benefits added as Part D by, 5, 120
Medicare Payment Advisory Commission (MedPAC), 74*n*4, 131, 137
fair compensation and, 57, 74*n*2
traditional Medicare compared to Medicare Advantage by, 67, 75*n*7
Medicare program, 20, 104
ACOs model in, 62–64
basics of, 117, 119–120
effect of, on new enrollees' health behaviors, 45, 46
future of private plans in, 133–137
as leader payment reform, 54–55, 59, 96
Part A as public hospitalization insurance, 5, 22, 61, 119–120, 121, 122
Part B as public outpatient/physician insurance, 5, 61, 120, 121, 122, 128
Part C as private (*see* Medicare Advantage plan)
Part D as private (*see* Prescription drugs)
spending for, 117, 118, 119, 121, 122, 127–134
supplements to, 118–119, 137–138
Medicare reform, 133–138
barriers to, 134
beneficiary incentives in, 136–137
Medigap reform included in, 137–138
premium support in, 135–136
provider payments, 133–134
shared-savings supplement in, 137
Medicare Shared Savings program
ACA and, 61
mathematical equations for fee-for-service payments to ACOs, 62–64, 68–69, 74–75*n*5, 76*n*6
Medigap program
help with copayments and deductibles in, 104, 128–129
as private addition to original Medicare program, 5, 119, 121, 124
reform, 137–138
standardized plans for, 122, 123*t*
Mediterranean diet, 23
MedPAC. *See* Medicare Payment Advisory Commission
Michigan, health insurance in, 43–44, 92
Moral hazard
ex ante, and substitute health care, 45, 46
health risks and insurance in, 2–3, 5, 105, 110–111, 125–126, 127
Mortality rates, 9, 47
projections of, in U.S. population pyramids, 10–11, 12*ff*–13*ff*
reduction in, and NIH research, 25–26

National Institutes of Health (NIH)
chronic disease research among, 16, 25–26
role in reducing health care costs, 24–26
Native Americans, exempted from ACA mandate, 83, 85*t*
Netherlands, medical spending in, 8*f*, 9*f*, 10*f*
New Zealand, medical spending in, 8*f*, 9*f*, 10*f*
NIH. *See* National Institutes of Health
Nursing home care, 104, 108
steps to avoid, 105–106, 110

Obama, Pres. Barack, reducing health care costs and, 4, 51, 75*n*9
Obesity, 24
BMI measurement and, 17–19, 18*f*, 19*f*, 31*n*8
epidemic of, and health care costs, 1, 20
European paradox and, 22–23
levels of education and, 28, 29*f*

Obesity, *cont.*
  prevention of, as food addiction through NIH research, 25–26
  quality of life and, 20, 21*ff*
  reduction of, and culture change, 23–24, 31*n*7
Oklahoma, workers' comp in, 92
Old Age and Survivors Insurance Fund, payroll tax and, 88
Omnibus Reconciliation Act, shift of Medigap regulation responsibility in, 121–122
Organisation for Economic Co-operation and Development (OECD) countries
  health care costs in, 1, 3, 6, 7–10, 8*f,* 9*f,* 10*f*
  student skills testing in, 26
Over-the-counter (OTC) drugs, 24, 47

Pain, poor lifestyle choices and, 24
Patient-Centered Outcomes Research Institute, mission and limitations of, 72–73, 97
Patient Protection and Affordable Care Act (ACA), 43
  ACO language in, 61, 74*n*4
  controversy about, 1, 103
  fewer uninsured as goal of, 43, 86, 97
  implementation of, 1, 82–86, 84*t*–85*t,* 108
  long-term care dropped from, 5, 103–104
  mandates with exemptions under, 1, 59, 67, 81, 82–82, 84*t*–85*t,* 103, 111
  Medicare cost reduction measures in, 83, 86, 96, 97
  more medical care than self-care with, 36, 38
  potential effects of, on social insurances, 4–5, 81–101
  reform of, 4, 11, 29–30, 51–55, 52*f*
  research institute established by, 72–73
Penalties, mandated in ACA, 82, 84*t*
Permanent partial disability (PPD), 92–93
Permanent total disability (PTD), 92–93
Personal responsibility, ACA mandate for, 1, 82–83, 84*t*–85*t,* 103, 111
Poland, medical spending in, 8*f,* 9*f,* 10*f*
Politics, as barrier to Medicare reform, 134
Population pyramids, 10–11, 12*f*–13*f*
  See also components, e.g., Elderly population; Working-age population
Portugal, medical spending in, 8*f,* 9, 9*f,* 10*f*
Postsecondary educational attainment, 26
  U.S. alcohol use by, 28, 30*f*
  U.S. obesity rates and, 28, 29*f*
  U.S. smokers with, 27*f,* 28
PPD. *See* Permanent partial disability
Preferred provider organizations (PPOs), Michigan BCBS among, 43
Prescription drugs, 5, 24, 47, 122
  insurance for, as Medicare Part D, 66, 69, 73, 76*n*13, 120, 136
  statins as, with substitution care effect, 46–47
Private health insurance, 60, 128
  ACOs models for, 64–65
  administrative loading and, 111
  BCBS as, 43–44, 64–65, 74*n*4
  future of, plans in Medicare, 133–137
  opportunities for, 104–105, 109–110
  role of, in Medicare, 5, 118–119, 120–124, 127–136
  See also Medicare Advantage plans; *and under* Prescription drugs, insurance for
Productivity, 24
  good health and, 1, 3, 37–38
PTD. *See* Permanent total disability

Quality care
  AQC and, 64–65, 69–70, 74*n*6, 133, 137
  competition in cost control for, 69, 135

Quality care, *cont.*
 trade-offs between cost and, 72, 73*f*, 74, 133
Quality of life, 1, 20, 21*ff*, 60

Rand Health Insurance Experiment, use of medical care in, and cost sharing, 125–126
Resource Based Relative Value Scale (RBRVS), payments to health care providers and, 56–57, 74*n*2
Retirement opportunities, 88, 96, 118
 ratio of those taking, to working-age population, 11, 12*ff*–13*ff*
Risk, 28, 39
 death, with chronic diseases, 18–19, 22, 23
 financial, and ACA protection against, 30–31, 74–75*n*5, 104
 health, and asymmetric information, 2–3, 110
 health, and competing models, 3–4, 35–44
 insurance design and, 2, 124–127
 long-term care, and elderly population, 5, 105, 112
Risk adjustment
 CLASS Act and, 107, 111
 Medicare Part C and, 68, 76*n*12
 Medicare Part D and, 69, 76*n*13
 methods for, 71, 122, 124, 130
 pools of enrollees in health insurance as, 61, 66–67, 70, 75*n*7
Risk aversion, 55
 decision making and, 39, 41–42
 insurance consumers attracted to, 111, 124
Ryan, U.S. House Speaker Paul, expansion of managed care and, 68, 75*n*9

Sebelius, HHS Secretary Kathleen, congressional charges to, 104, 108
Self-care, 2
 empirical papers on, 45–47
 procyanadin consumption in, 20, 31*n*6
 sole use of, or in combination with medical care, 3–4, 40–44, 47–48
Silver tsunami, 11
Sleep apnea, as chronic disease, 19
Slovak Republic, medical spending in, 8*f*, 9, 9*f*, 10*f*
Social insurance programs. *See specific types, i.e.,* Social Security system; Disability insurance; Workers' compensation
Social Security system
 benefits paid by, 88, 111, 113
 payments into, 86, 88
Social Security Disability Insurance (SSDI), 86–88, 88–91, 88*f*, 111
 spending on, 53, 53*f*, 118
South Korea, medical spending in, 8*f*, 9*f*, 10*f*
Spain, medical spending in, 8*f*, 9*f*, 10*f*
SSDI. *See* Social Security Disability Insurance
Supplemental Security Income (SSI), 86, 87–88, 89*f*, 90
Supplementary Medical Insurance program, 120
Sweden, medical spending in, 7, 8*f*, 9*f*, 10*f*
Switzerland, medical spending in, 8*f*, 9*f*, 10*f*

Tanzania
 EPI and maternal care complementarity in, 45–46
Tax Equity and Fiscal Responsibility Act, Medicare Part C and, 122
Taxes, 86
 employer subsidy on, 29, 43
 Medicare and Medicaid funding through, 20, 29, 88, 118
 payroll, as Part A funders, 88, 120
Technological improvements, health care spending and, 117
Temporary total disability (TTD) benefits, initial, 92
Terry, Surgeon General Luther, smoking report and, 17, 27–28, 27*f*
Texas, workers' comp in, 92, 95

Time horizons, 110
  internal discount rate and, 26, 31*n*9
  long-term care insurance and, 112, 113–114
Tobacco use, 3
  as actual cause of death, 15–17, 15*f,* 20, 22
  cigarette smoking in, 16–17, 16*f,* 30*n*2
  levels of education and, 27–28, 27*f*
  prevention of, addiction through NIH research, 25–26
Trade-offs
  between cost and quality, 72, 73*f,* 74
  between risk and return or income, 39
TTD. *See* Temporary total disability

UN. *See* United Nations
Uncertainty, 6, 88
  health care and, 38–44, 104
  health insurance choices and, 3–4
  health status, and insurance, 2, 39, 55
  prudence as concept in, 41–42
United Kingdom, 22
  medical spending in, 7, 8*f,* 9*f,* 10*f*
United Nations (UN), EPI implementation in developing countries, 45–46
United States (U.S.), 22
  aging population of, 6, 53
  health and medical spending in, 7–9, 8*f,* 9*f,* 10*f,* 51–55, 52*f,* 53*f,* 74*n*1
  infant mortality and life expectancy in, 8–9, 36
U.S. Congress, 134
  advisers to, 56–57, 67, 74*n*2, 83
  CBO oversight for, 52–53, 74*n*1, 83, 103, 108–109
  House of Representatives proposals, 67–68, 75*n*9
  Senate committees, 103–104
U.S. Dept. of Health and Human Services (HHS)
  activities of, 104, 108
U.S. government agencies, 24, 25
  cash and counseling programs by, 106, 108
  program budgets, 108–109, 117, 124, 130
U.S. law and legislation
  health care in, 1, 5, 83, 110, 122
  state-level regulations, 121–122
U.S. Supreme Court, rulings, 83, 103

Wages, indemnity benefits and, 92–93, 93*f*
War on chronic diseases, 25
War on drugs, 20, 22
Weight-loss products, health care spending and, 24
Workers' compensation insurance, 111
  nature and purpose of, 4–5, 81, 92–93, 93*f*
  potential effects of ACA on, 81–82, 94–98
  See also Disability insurance
Working-age population, 95, 96
  CLASS program and, 103, 105, 110, 111
  ratio of, *vs.* retirees, 11, 12*ff*–13*ff*
  See also Labor force

Young population, 95, 119
  See also Population pyramids

Zambia, EPI and maternal care complementarity in, 45–46
Zimbabwe, EPI and maternal care complementarity in, 45–46

About the Institute

The W.E. Upjohn Institute for Employment Research is a nonprofit research organization devoted to finding and promoting solutions to employment-related problems at the national, state, and local levels. It is an activity of the W.E. Upjohn Unemployment Trustee Corporation, which was established in 1932 to administer a fund set aside by Dr. W.E. Upjohn, founder of The Upjohn Company, to seek ways to counteract the loss of employment income during economic downturns.

The Institute is funded largely by income from the W.E. Upjohn Unemployment Trust, supplemented by outside grants, contracts, and sales of publications. Activities of the Institute comprise the following elements: 1) a research program conducted by a resident staff of professional social scientists; 2) a competitive grant program, which expands and complements the internal research program by providing financial support to researchers outside the Institute; 3) a publications program, which provides the major vehicle for disseminating the research of staff and grantees, as well as other selected works in the field; and 4) an Employment Management Services division, which manages most of the publicly funded employment and training programs in the local area.

The broad objectives of the Institute's research, grant, and publication programs are to 1) promote scholarship and experimentation on issues of public and private employment and unemployment policy, and 2) make knowledge and scholarship relevant and useful to policymakers in their pursuit of solutions to employment and unemployment problems.

Current areas of concentration for these programs include causes, consequences, and measures to alleviate unemployment; social insurance and income maintenance programs; compensation; workforce quality; work arrangements; family labor issues; labor-management relations; and regional economic development and local labor markets.